More, Please

More, Please

On Food, Fat, Bingeing, Longing, and the Lust for "Enough"

Emma Specter

HARPER

An Imprint of HarperCollins*Publishers*

HarperCollins books may be purchased for educational, business, or sales promotional use. For information, please email the Special Markets Department at SPsales@harpercollins.com.

FIRST EDITION

Title page art courtesy of Shutterstock / Alex Farias

Library of Congress Cataloging-in-Publication Data has been applied for.

ISBN 978-0-06-327837-0

24 25 26 27 28 LBC 5 4 3 2 1

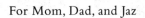

For Mom, Dad, and Jaz

"The first sin was a woman eating."

—Ruth Gibbs, "Faithful Food"

"What nourishes me destroys me."

—Leslie from *America's Next Top Model* Cycle 6's
lower-abdomen tattoo

CONTENTS

INTRODUCTION

I'm in my bed. I'm always in my bed, always sweating an imprint of myself onto the sheets, always letting crumbs and streaks of grease land on the once-pristine white duvet cover I never take the time to roll up and off the mattress.

I'm eating. I'm always eating. It's pizza this time, drunkenly ordered off Seamless from the back of the Lyft home from the bar after yet another mildly disappointing night out. It doesn't taste good or bad, not after the first few bites. Once I get into my groove, each slice is a blissful nothing, the swallowing of the crust a hard push against my throat that is quickly mellowed by the next still-hot, pliant bite of cheese and sauce dissolving in my mouth.

Nothing much happened tonight—nothing more than any other Saturday night in my recent past: my friends and I gathered for drinks at someone's apartment before heading to the club. I wore a dress I thought I liked that turned out to fit me wrong, gaping open at the chest every time I reached my arms up to dance. I struck out with a girl I'd been eyeing across the dance floor, a girl whose name I never quite learned but whose implied rejection stung nonetheless. It's these nights—the nights where I wade into the gap between my rosy perception of my New York life and its actual, lived reality—that most reliably lead to a binge. Sometimes they don't, but when they do, it always feels inevitable, as though no other outcome was remotely possible.

Every binge is the same. That's not true, of course; I've binged in the darkened kitchen of my childhood home, in my best friend's bathroom, in my dorm bed, in a shabby Russian hostel, in the economy lounge at Paris's Charles de Gaulle Airport, in a tiny LA one-bedroom shared with a roommate and in more places than I can possibly list. Each of those separate binges was precipitated by its own set of circumstances, but there's something flattening about the act of binge eating itself—of shoving food furtively into my mouth as quickly and passively as I can—that makes each individual binge feel tethered to the one before it, like beads strung on a common thread. *This is who I am*, my brain dully reminds me as I eat, and when I'm mid-binge, there on my bed, junk-food wrappers and paper bags surrounding me like confetti from the world's loneliest parade, I have trouble steeling myself enough to fight off the thought. It's so much easier to sigh, give in, sprint to the kitchen for a spoon or a fork, lock the bedroom door, and let the tide of numb eating carry me out.

The way it works, roughly, is this: something happens, as big as a breakup or a firing or as small as a tiff with a friend or a favorite earring lost, and an hour or a day or a week later, I start to feel the gnawing, seductive urge to binge. Not that I'd ever call it "bingeing" in my head, mind you; when the binge is still ahead of me, rather than a *fait accompli*, I tell myself I'll keep it to one croissant, one full-fat iced latte, one Pop-Tart from the office kitchen, one "forbidden" food item to fix my bad mood. I probably don't have to tell you that it's never just one, and what's "forbidden" quickly becomes unprecious by way of glassy-eyed repetition.

The primary condition of my bingeing has always been solitude—solitude, and a desire to no longer be. The "purest" pleasure I can liken it to is the feeling of swimming way out in the ocean, the way I used to when I lived in Los Angeles, driving out to Malibu and letting my rusty Subaru bake in the early-morning sun while I dove beneath the waves. I'd breaststroke and crawl my way out, far out, past the buoys, past the point where any sensible lifeguard would have blown their whistle, and then I'd float, suspended in salt, my limbs pale and blissfully irrelevant beneath the dark, deep water. What I was doing was dangerous, I knew, and I eventually stopped making a habit of swimming out quite so far, but I feel like I return to that weight-less, consequence-free place in the water every time I binge. When I binge, I'm not possessed of a body, not weighed down by breasts and hips and stretch-marked flesh; I am just a hand moving fork to mouth, two eyes fluttering and slowly closing to sleep off the worst of the food-induced nausea and indigestion.

I first became aware of Lee Price's "Women and Food" series, in which the New York–based artist captures herself in the act of binge eating, in a 2014 article for a popular online women's publication. My initial reaction was to recoil from the article's framing, which seemed to present binge eating as "something we all do, right?"—a cheeky foible along the lines of Bridget Jones's penchant for cigarettes and wine units. When I saw Price's paintings, though, the thought came to me unbidden: *Oh, no. Nobody's supposed to see this.* In the paintings, Price is always alone, usually in her bed or in a bathtub, ringed with garlands of Twinkies and Lay's and Chinese takeout; in *Jelly Donuts* (2010), the most striking image of the series, she's lying on a white bed in a pristine white tank top and panties, eyes fixed upward, one hand to her mouth, the scarlet filling of a jelly donut staining her midsection like a gunshot wound. All the days and nights I'd filled with food, all the time I'd spent sweating and groaning atop my mattress— because binge eating, whatever else it might be, is intensely physical, even as it seems to momentarily anesthetize the body— Price had trained a floodlight on them, and I could neither look too closely nor look away.

"My use of the bird's-eye view gets interpreted as a voyeurism thing or a God's eye view a lot—it's neither. It's the subject looking down on herself—observing herself in the act of the compulsive behavior, being completely aware of what she is doing but unable to stop," Price told *The Other Journal* in a 2011 interview. All these years later, I've still never heard a better description of what I am, what I do to myself; I know what I'm doing, know the thick-tongued, crusty-eyed regret I'll wake to the next morning, yet I can't seem to will myself to stop. There are no crazy stories to characterize my addiction, no adrenaline-spiking capers or wild nights out: There's just me, lying oily-stomached and prone in the aftermath of a binge, just like Price in her 2008 painting *Asleep*, which shows her curled up on her side in bed with her eyes closed, pastel-iced cupcakes fanned out all around her. It's a beautiful image, in the classical sense—Price could be Ophelia in the famous Sir John Everett Millais painting, eyes unseeing as her body is carried downstream—but the empty wrapper by her head and the streak of frosting on her knee are the clues that tell the real story to those of us in the know, those of us who look at a supermarket cereal aisle or a Burger King TV commercial and see our own slow-motion undoing.

Like Price, my tastes in binge food are wholly and unreservedly American. If it's sweet, salty, or of a color not found in nature, chances are good I've binged on it at least once. As a child growing up in Italy, I lusted after Oreos, cramming them in my mouth hand over fist whenever friends from the US would bring them over in their checked luggage, waiting for my parents to be suitably distracted before absconding to my bedroom with a full sleeve. Cheez-Its were my college go-to, the big party-sized boxes from the Snack Foods aisle of the Kroger a few miles off campus, their razor-sharp edges turning to a neon-orange mush in my mouth. During my semester abroad in St. Petersburg, I stayed in my room for days at a time to avoid the bone-chilling frost, foraying out only to buy economy-sized tubs of imported Ben & Jerry's marked up to an absurd price. In Los Angeles, newly postgrad, I favored massive rings of glazed doughnuts from the bakery down the street from my apartment. In Brooklyn, I'd eat one polite slice of the homemade pizza my roommates spent hours concocting before cracking, my taste for carbs activated, and consuming a large Papa John's pie (plus cheesy bread) alone after midnight once everyone was asleep.

I've consumed all of these foods, and more, many times in my life, often joyfully and without turning them into "binge food," which is exactly what makes binge eating disorder B.E.D., to those regrettably in the know—so complex. The food you tearfully shove down at 3 a.m. and stand over the sink trying futilely to vomit up might be the same food you enjoy at a convivial brunch with friends, savoring the taste on your tongue between hearty laughter and sips of coffee. *It's not what you're eating, it's what's eating you*, the conventional wisdom holds, and it's true that Cheez-Its and Papa John's themselves are value-neutral. They're, well . . . "just food," and relatively cheap food at that, food that a majority of Americans can actually find at their local supermarket or corner store and afford to feed to their families. When I'm sad, or bored, or lonely, or tired, or feeling nothing at all, though, these everyday snacks turn into my own personal bogeymen, representing my darkest impulses to stuff myself, gorge myself, hurt myself. Detangling the foods themselves from the ways in which I've used them to self-harm is a task that might take me the rest of my life to accomplish.

If I'm making my binge eating sound pretty, succumbing to the desire to make my addiction poetic in the grand tradition of Ernest Hemingway and John Berryman, let me assure you that it's not. I wish it were—I wish there were a literary or artistic tradition formed around binge eating, if only so I didn't feel quite so aberrant—but there's nothing pretty about the sickening, ever so slightly freeing realization of, *Oh fuck, I could eat right now*, followed shortly by *I am going to eat right now*. There's nothing lovely about the sweatpants-clad, eyes-downcast shuffle to the grocery store for a cart overflowing with cookies and chips, and there's nothing romantic about the amount of money I've spent ordering cartons of freezer-hardened ice cream and grease-puddled boxes of pizza on the food-delivery apps I pride myself on not using when I'm what I call "normal"—i.e., when I'm not bingeing. When I'm bingeing, I tell myself, the rules do not apply; not just the punishing food rules I've lived by since I was old enough for my first Weight Watchers stint, but also the rules of social engagement, of politeness, of active presence in whatever space I'm required to inhabit.

Binge eating disorder has a complex history, but it's one that doesn't date back all that far in the American imagination. In 1959, psychiatrist Albert Stunkard published a paper titled "Eating Patterns and Obesity," in which he described the phenomenon of "the eating binge, in which large amounts of food are consumed in an orgiastic manner at irregular intervals." Stunkard also coined the term "night eating syndrome" in the same paper, though he later clarified that binge eating didn't necessarily have to happen at night; today, night eating syndrome (NES) is classified as its own eating disorder, one that affects about one in ten people who have obesity.

While Stunkard's paper introduced the concept of binge eating into the medical lexicon, it wasn't until 1987 that the American Psychological Association (APA) first mentioned the disease in its Diagnostic and Statistical Manual of Mental Disorders (DSM). At the time, binge eating was merely referred to as one facet of bulimia; it took another seven years for binge eating to be formally listed in the DSM, though its inclusion was still maintained as a feature of "eating disorder not otherwise specified." Finally, in 2013, a revised edition of the DSM declared binge eating to be its own disorder, allowing its treatment to be covered under many insurance plans and codifying a series of criteria that included "feelings of distress relating to eating behaviors" and "frequency of bingeing at least once a week for three or more months." Shame and self-recrimination are quite literally built into the diagnostic framework of binge eating disorder, and any method of healing that doesn't proactively address the sources of those feelings seems to be treating the symptom instead of the disease.

When I attended my first twelve-step "food group" meeting, I was asked to make a list of all the ways my addiction had hurt the people around me. Everything else we'd talked about in the meeting—the food fixation, the shame, the physical and emotional discomfort—hit home, but that one stupefied me. *What am I supposed to do, send a letter of apology to the girl from summer camp whose bag of Goldfish I secretly ate when we were eleven?* I wondered to myself, all too ready to make fun of the program (because God forbid I actually took it seriously—who would I be then?). Bingeing hadn't made me cheat on a partner, or commit grand theft auto, or physically harm anyone; sure, I'd lied in order to enable my addiction, but those lies were of the "I can't make it to the party because I have a migraine" variety. Victimless crimes, or so I thought.

Today, I can see that the plans I canceled had people on the other end, people who wanted to see me. The money I spent could have been put toward trips with my best friends, nice gifts for family Christmases instead of random crap I'd rush-purchased at the airport, donations to causes I cared about; anything but binge meals I'd devour at once and instantly regret. Even the food I used as a security blanket was usually delivered to me by precariously employed gig-economy workers making, on average, far less than the hourly federal minimum wage. Food has always helped me shut the world out, and when I realized that fact, I was suffused with shame and regret. Those feelings led, predictably, to more bingeing. Slowly, though, over the course of many binges and stutter-stepped next-day recoveries, I began to see that the person I was hurting the most with my addiction was, well . . . me. Somehow, I'd never thought to count myself.

Chapter 1

WATCH

For as long as I can remember, my mother has been beautiful. The "conventional" kind of beautiful, too, though her personality has always been self-deprecating enough to let you forget it—wide-set eyes, straight nose, full mouth, blond bob. When I was sixteen, I went hunting through drawers for batteries and came across a stack of my mom's press passes from the beginning of her journalism career. A late-twenties version of my mom stared defiantly out at me from the laminated square in my hand, the symmetry of her face unmarred by her wedge haircut and oh-so-'80s suit, and instead of being awed or nostalgic, I felt panicked. Suddenly, I was all too aware of my own aquiline nose, my thin lips, the fleshly spread of my thighs in their cutoff jean shorts; the splendor of my mother in black-and-white suddenly felt like an inheritance I was squandering, a repudiation in and of itself.

Our mothers tend to loom large in our minds and in the ways we move through the world, whether we want them to or not, and for daughters, the urge to compare can be irresistible, even inescapable. After all, how many of us are single because our mothers married young, or stay-at-home moms because our mothers worked, or dog owners because our mothers hated pets? When it comes to body image, that tendency toward comparison can be particularly toxic. I'm one of the lucky ones, in that my mother has never outright told me to lose weight, but there's so much that can be communicated with a meaningful look or the subtle raise of an eyebrow over dinner; these days, I consider us close, but for years, it felt like my mother and I were tethered to each other by an invisible umbilical cord of judgment.

It's not lost on me that my very first experiences of physical satiety came at the expense of my mother's sanity. During my babyhood, the "breast is best" philosophy prevailed, with few nonjudgmental resources available to mothers who chose to bottle-feed, and my mother dutifully learned to feed me with her body. She's always painted a rosy portrait of my babyhood, constantly telling me how cute I was—"People would always try to pinch your cheeks!"—and how much she adored toting me around Central Park in my stroller and breastfeeding me on demand, but I still can't help thinking of her jolting awake for endless 3:00 a.m. feedings, doing her best to supply nourishment to a tiny, helpless baby who always seemed to be hungry.

To truly understand the origins of my eating disorder—and, indeed, much of America's love-hate relationship with food—requires a return to the very beginning of taste: childhood. My family moved around the world for my parents' work, with the three of us leaving New York when I was six months old and living in three different countries before my ninth birthday. Unfortunately, all that exposure to new foods didn't embolden me to actually try many of them, despite my parents' prodding; there were certain meals I loved, like—improbably—fried calamari, and I'd charm the adults by ordering a basket of them "for the table" at meals out, but I pretty much avoided any that I didn't. My bland palate was forged early, and I refused borscht and herring in Russia, Parmesan cheese and red sauce in Italy, instead subsisting on plain pasta and rice. One of the happiest memories of my childhood was the day a Dunkin' Donuts opened in Rome; somewhere in a leather-bound photo album there exist photos of me astride my father's shoulders in my cow-print leggings and pink sweatshirt, jubilantly cramming perfectly round circles of frosted dough into my mouth.

When we moved, for a third and final time, back to New York, I joyfully discovered that the bodegas lining Broadway all sold candy bars for cheap, and that school was a bountiful resource for what my teachers called "snacks" (a concept I'd been unfamiliar with in Italy, where conventional wisdom held that food was for mealtimes). There were Cheez-Its in little Dixie cups, a veritable Noah's ark of animal crackers, and, on classmates' birthdays, cupcakes, store-bought from Yura on Madison, and thick with pink and yellow frosting. We arrived in New York a few months before the Twin Towers fell, and my memories of that time are of fear and sweetness combined; the photos of people in gas masks that grimaced crudely up at me from the front pages of magazines adorning stoops on the walk to school, the lightness of sugar and pastry evaporating on my tongue as we celebrated the momentous occasion of Emily C. turning eight.

Food meant comfort for everyone that year, with high school girls and grandfathers and investment bankers alike turning up at the doors of fire stations around the city with trays of lasagna and sheets of cookies. In her memoir *Save Me the Plums*, former *Gourmet* editor in chief Ruth Reichl recalls putting the magazine's eight kitchens to use dishing up vats of chili for the firefighters at Ground Zero, writing, "We were attempting to snatch hope from the rubble of our broken city. And food was the perfect way to do it." Maybe it was around 9/11 that I first learned to associate food with safety, but really, doesn't every child do that? The very word *more*—which many kids learn to deploy early—conjures an expansiveness, a promise of infinite pleasure to come that a three-year-old doesn't yet know to question. The deal is the same on any playground in America—"Stop crying/ put that down/be good, and you'll get a treat"—but how does it work when you're old enough to know where Mom keeps the cookies? What happens to "being good" when the power to reward or punish yourself with food is in your hands alone?

As the constitutionally anxious only child of two hardworking journalist parents, I learned to self-soothe with food early and often upon our return to New York, taking refuge in leftover Halloween candy on late work nights and gratefully accepting my babysitter Nadia's offers of Domino's on TV-centric Friday evenings. Am I a binge eater now because of Reese's Peanut Butter Cups and takeout pizza eaten quietly alone in front of

Lizzie McGuire, without my parents around or the clatter of siblings to distract me? Maybe, to some degree. But if that were wholly accurate, wouldn't every only child whose parents worked long hours have binge eating disorder? And, conversely, wouldn't every child who had a *Leave It to Beaver* upbringing have a sterling, spectacularly unemotional relationship with food?

We know that's not true, yet it can't be denied that many of our disordered attachments (to food, as well as to a wealth of other vices) begin in youth, particularly in the United States; as Karen Le Billon wrote of having her thoroughly American food and child-rearing instincts thrown into question by a move to France when her daughters were young in her 2012 book *French Kids Eat Everything*, "I was using food as a reward, a bribe, a toy, a distraction and a substitute for discipline. The problem, from the French perspective, was that I was teaching my kids to use food as a response to emotional needs, which have little to no nutritional basis." The "French perspective" might condemn Le Billon and other parents for this, but it makes perfect sense to me even after just a few scant summers of nannying. When a child is crying or upset or acting out, the natural urge is to offer up anything you can to make them stop. It's no wonder so many new parents torture themselves over breastfeeding versus formula-feeding; what could be a more weighty responsibility than being solely responsible for the care and feeding of a small human being?

There's little that we, as a society, love to do more than shame parents—and, more specifically, mothers—for the way they bring up their children, particularly when those parents happen to deviate even slightly from the straight, white, happily married nuclear-suburban "ideal." That's part of why I'm now hesitant to find fault with either of my parents, but particularly my mother, for what I now know to call my eating disorder. Did my mom make frequent comments about wanting to lose weight and fill our house with the faux junk food that was ever-present in the diet-centric early 2000s? Yes, but she was the busy working mother of a tween daughter; the odds that she was going to be able to instill a wholly positive body image in me anywhere, let alone in image-obsessed aughts Manhattan, were not good.

Leslie Sim, a child psychologist and clinical director of the Mayo Clinic's eating disorders program, told *USA Today* in 2013 that "moms are probably the most important influence on a daughter's body image." If that statement holds true (as, in my anecdotal experience, it does), it's easy to imagine how much pressure mothers around the world might feel to model a constructive relationship with food that they simply don't know how to kick-start. Most daughters out there can likely attest to the truth of Sim's statement, and I certainly had no small share of clashes with my mom in department-store dressing rooms and chain restaurants over the years, but as an adult, it seems inconceivable to me that we expect a generation of women warped by decades' worth of media-reinforced fatphobia to raise children who are any less—to put it frankly—fucked up about bodies and food.

My mother was born in 1955, the year the first McDonald's franchise opened in the United States; meanwhile, every model who graced the cover of American *Vogue* that year was impossibly lean. My mom and her compatriots made it through decades of fad diets, from the SlimFast revolution of the late 1970s to the cabbage-soup program that must have led to an awful lot of gastrointestinal distress in the 1980s. In 1993, the year my mom gave birth to me, Jazzercise had taken over, along with its very own diet plan that ditched calorie counting in favor of a rainbow-hued chart that let you know which foods were "okay" to eat. Is it any wonder that all of that messaging—not to mention a fraught relationship with her own mother, my grandmother, who'd been raised eating the twentieth-century equivalent of Oliver Twist's gruel in an Italian orphanage and who deployed "fat" readily as a barb throughout her life—didn't adequately prepare her to raise a wholly body-confident daughter?

In my teens, years in which I assumed the oh-so-predictable stance of blaming my parents for absolutely everything, I grimly deduced that it was my mom's fault I was so screwed up about food. After all, if she hadn't let me quit the softball team at ten, hadn't allowed me to try Weight Watchers (or, as it's now known, "WW") at twelve, hadn't talked so much about wanting to drop ten pounds as I approached my teens, maybe I would be just fine now, capable of eating dessert without guilt and trying on swimsuits sans shame. Why couldn't she have raised me in the kind of all-organic, body-positive Valhalla in which I swore to bring up my own children someday, walking around the house naked whenever the mood struck and picking fresh greens from the garden as desired? (Did my self-pitying reverie take into account the fact that I had never known actual material scarcity, food-based or otherwise, in my seventeen years on the planet? Or that I'd soon be off to sulk and write feminist blog diatribes at a private liberal arts college paid for in full by the work my parents were so busy doing throughout my childhood? It did not.)

Luckily, early in college, I crossed paths with a gifted therapist who was simply unable—or unwilling—to stomach my wallowing. She told me bluntly: "Listen, you were probably going to be addicted to something. You should be glad it's food." I didn't know what to do with that comment for a long time, but looking back on it now, I marvel at its aptness. I come from a lineage of drinkers on one side and gamblers on the other, and while much of my extended family has been able to avoid the worst consequences of full-blown substance dependency through a mixture of privilege and sheer good luck, there's no denying that some degree of addiction is in my genes. I was also diagnosed with clinical depression at nineteen, a mental illness that is frequently associated with higher rates of obesity and binge eating disorder—my queerness, too, puts me at an increased risk for any number of eating disorders.

My aunt Flavia—my mother's little sister—was twenty-five when I was born, and has always functioned as my bonus big sister. We've both always been larger-bodied than my mother ever has been, something we're reminded of at family gatherings every time my mom serves up platefuls of freshly sizzling bacon to my lanky male cousins and offers Flavia and me peeled clementines instead. (We always meet each other's eyes, brows raised, before diving in for a handful of the boys' bacon.) Flavia's and my eye rolls over my mom's not-so-subtle messaging aside, dieting was always the way in which my mom and Flavia bonded, and the way I learned to bond with them, too. Throughout my childhood, Flavia would show up at my mom's apartment and immediately be handed a coffee or a Coke Zero before throwing a load of laundry into the washer and settling down in the kitchen to chat. "You look good" was always the salutation served with Flavia's drink, setting her up for the spike: "Ugh, no I don't, I'm so fat" would come the reply, or sometimes, "Thanks! I'm trying Atkins again."

As I got older and moved out, I, too, learned to show up at my mom's with an armful of dirty laundry and an opening salvo of self-deprecation: "Do you have skim for the coffee? None of my jeans fit, I hate myself," I'd announce dramatically, performing my role in our twisted little Greek chorus of communal insecurity. On some level, I wonder if we were quick to judge ourselves out loud so that nobody else would feel tempted—after all, our broader extended family, the men in particular, weren't the type to spare our feelings if we showed up for Christmas having gained a few. When I restarted Weight Watchers in earnest my senior year of college, I'd come home bearing mind-blowing calorie facts about movie-theater popcorn and restaurant nachos. When I lost weight, then kept on losing it, after a postgrad move to LA, I not-so-secretly delighted in my mom's mix of pride and concern over my thinness, showing off my lack of appetite like I was displaying a dazzling new magic trick: "No dinner for me, thanks, I'm not that hungry."

One of the very first genuine representations of binge eating disorder in popular culture that I ever saw just so happened to feature a mother who binged, instilling in me both peace (okay, so I wasn't the only person in the world who did this) and terror (would I still be like this by the time I had kids?). Frankie Shaw's *SMILF* ran for two seasons on Showtime, and while the series wasn't perfect, on-screen or off—Shaw was investigated for on-set misconduct claims, and the series was ultimately canceled soon after its second season aired—the story that it endeavored to tell about women, parenting, class, addiction, and food was profoundly ambitious. In the pilot episode, single mother Bridgette (Shaw) finds herself home alone with her sleeping child, in a shame spiral after masturbating to photos of her ex-boyfriend's new girlfriend. To the strains of Beirut's "Santa Fe," she tucks her baby in, puts on her sneakers, and sprints to a nearby grocery store, filling her arms with chips, cookies, and brownies, then covering her tracks by telling an old hookup she's just run into that she's buying snacks for her son's birthday party.

Back at home, Bridgette binges, then texts her old flame to come over for sex, quickly making herself throw up in the sink before he arrives. She binges and purges several more times throughout the series, suggesting that her diagnosis might be bulimia, not just binge eating disorder; her best friend Eliza (Raven Goodwin) is a woman she met in her local chapter of a loosely defined "food group" for people who suffer from various problems relating to disordered eating. Eliza is frequently shown to be in a vicious and all-too-relatable cycle of stress eating over her demanding father's expectations, then panicking over how to hide her weight gain from him in what Bridgette refers to as "shame clothes." For her part, Bridgette binges and purges when she feels particularly lonely and out of control over her single status, poverty, and history of sexual abuse, while her own over-bearing mother Tutu (Rosie O'Donnell) uses food alternately as a cudgel and an entreaty, first pushing Bridgette away, then beckoning her back over for a home-cooked dinner.

The mothers and daughters of *SMILF* made me feel uncomfortably seen when the show premiered in 2017, in a way I didn't yet have the language to express. I'd seen plenty of women who looked like Shaw—thin, white, conventionally attractive—eat emotionally on TV shows like *Friends* and *Will and Grace*, but those were sitcoms that played on the absurdity of women who looked like Courteney Cox or Debra Messing downing an entire cheesecake. *SMILF* was different in that it stayed trained on its protagonist once the binge food was cleared away, refusing to lighten the mood with a laugh track as Bridgette stood up in her dingy apartment and retched into the sink. Though my experience is worlds away from Bridgette's, I, too, know what lengths I'll go to in order to procure binge food for myself, and I know how readily I'll lie about it if anyone questions me.

The child Bridgette is raising solo on *SMILF* is a boy, but she still worries aloud that he'll grow up to have an eating disorder (as, in fact, 1.6 percent of American boys between the ages of nine and ten do). When I rewatch *SMILF* and note Bridgette's furtive approach to food, maybe it's a sign of growth that I no longer see myself; instead, I see a young mother struggling to provide better for her child, doing what she can to seek help for her eating disorder while occasionally reverting to the self-soothing method that comes most naturally to her. Would it, in fact, be Bridgette's "fault" if her son Larry did grow up to have an eating disorder?

The internet is awash in "success stories" about mother-child pairs shedding vast amounts of weight together, with *Women's Health* running an "exclusive" online interview in 2014 with a mother and daughter who lost a combined seventy-four pounds in one hundred days. (It's worth noting that the Centers for Disease Control and Prevention recommend a weight loss rate of no more than two pounds per week, which casts the speed of this slim down and others like it in a somewhat more alarming light.) We're meant to marvel at the cross-generational willpower evidenced in stories like these, but all I think about when I read them is what the mothers and daughters on display might have felt about how their relationships might have grown had they jointly discovered sea kayaking instead—or puzzles, or bread baking, or volunteer meal delivery, or *Selling Sunset.*

In an ideal world, nobody would become a parent without some measure of compassion and appreciation for their own body, but in the world we actually inhabit, nothing could be further from the truth. In a 2018 study, published in the *International Journal of Eating Disorders,* researchers surveyed 581 parents of children ages nine to fifteen and found that 76 percent of the parents insulted their own bodies in front of their children, and 43.6 percent talked negatively about their children's bodies. Unsurprisingly, the children of the parents in the latter group were more likely to engage in "binge eating, secretive eating or other disordered behaviors," raising the question: How do we give parents the tools they need to help protect their kids against eating disorders without further contributing to a culture of mom shaming that so often falls along racial, ethnic, and socioeconomic lines?

One thing that is frequently left out of the cultural conversation about binge eating—to the extent that there is one—is its sheer, widespread accessibility as far as addictions and substance dependencies go. Yes, food costs money, but generally less so than alcohol or drugs, and even more significantly, you can binge eat while still remaining lucid enough to show up for work or watch your kid. "In my experience, certain populations of women are most at risk for compulsive overeating. These are the women who are caretakers, whose life work is nurturing others. Nurses, for example, are notorious for having goodies in their nursing stations and eating when they are overworked and tired," wrote Mary Pipher in her 1994 bestseller *Reviving Ophelia*, and although not everything from that book holds up (she goes on to say that it's "virtually impossible in America to be heavy and feel good about oneself"—I disagree, to say the least), the caretaking part makes sense to me. In an increasingly "hustle culture"–driven society, where the word "binge" is cleverly deployed to get you to stream a TV show or order dinner from Seamless—"Hey, we get it," the millennial-written ad copy seems to winkingly say—how are parents supposed to recognize that they have a genuine problem, much less shield their kids from developing it, too?

I've always hoped to be a mother, but it's taken a long time for me to actually voice that desire out loud, due to a mix of low self-esteem (who would ever want to have a baby with *me*?)

and internalized anxiety about my own sexuality that set in long before I officially came out at twenty-four (it was hard enough for straight women to get pregnant, so how would *I* ever manage to pull it off?). These days, I'm open about wanting kids; I'm not ready yet, but I tell myself that all the things I fear about becoming a mom will eventually pass, or at least lessen to the point where they don't feel like cons that outweigh the pros of parenthood. One thing that still flummoxes me, though, is what my therapist and I call "the body thing." How will I manage to raise children who feel good, or at least okay, about food and their bodies, when I'm still regularly battling my own eating disorder with what often feels like every ounce of strength I can summon?

Intellectually, I know you don't have to be eating disorder–free, or in any way "done" with the often-lifelong project of attaining stable mental health, to be a good parent. (And who decides what "good" is, anyway? Personally, I'm partial to British pediatrician and psychotherapist Donald Winnicott's theory of the "good-enough mother," whom he describes as one who "starts off with an almost complete adaptation to her infant's needs, and as time proceeds she adapts less and less completely, gradually, according to the infant's growing ability to deal with her failure." Getting progressively worse at something and calling it a parenting technique? Sign me up!) All that said, I'm terrified that my own internalized fatphobia and disordered eating will infect my child's psyche, even if I ban Barbies from the household and always make sure to pack a well-rounded school lunch.

I still think about the way Zadie Smith characterized female self-hatred in her 2005 novel *On Beauty*, describing it as seeping in "with every draught in the house; people brought it home on their shoes, they breathed it in off their newspapers. There was no way to control it." In theory, this idea should be somewhat comforting, allowing all prospective mothers to accept the probability that they will inevitably, at some point, fail in protecting their daughters against bodily disgust. Still, I pray that I'll be able to conquer my lifelong binge eating disorder by the time I have kids, thus ushering them into a home in which food represents only joy or fuel, never failure. Unfortunately, the "get better by thirty-five"—or thirty-two, or forty, or wherever it happens, if it happens—speaks directly to the eating disorder–addled part of my brain, seductively cooing to me that I don't *really* need to get better until I'm responsible for someone other than myself. So often, those struggling with addiction or compulsion are urged to get better "for your kids," or for their parents, or for some other external force, but what does that say about our intrinsic value? Aren't we worthy of healing for our own sake?

In her 2022 book *Fat Talk: Parenting in the Age of Diet Culture*, journalist Virginia Sole-Smith—who has written extensively about the ways in which fatphobia and weight stigma can affect kids—notes that not being fat as a child left her largely unprepared to handle the struggles that came with gaining weight as a young adult. "I was a thin kid once, too," recalls Sole-Smith in the introduction to *Fat Talk*, writing: "I remember reveling in the knowledge that adults in my life envied my body, which, until college, I felt mostly good about. And then my body changed." (*And then my body changed*—a horror story in five words, one likely to elicit a shiver of recognition from anyone who's ever gone through puberty.) Sole-Smith is now the mother of two girls, and while she spent years attempting to detangle weight and worth in both her writing and her personal life, it took a frightening medical emergency for her to finally break up with diet culture for good.

"My older daughter was born with this rare congenital heart defect and she totally stopped eating as a baby, so we had this really traumatic time of helping her navigate a lot of surgeries and learning how to eat again. That was kind of my 'come to Jesus' moment with diet culture," Sole-Smith tells me, adding: "I had come up through women's magazines and spent all this time trying to justify my work as a feminist but also writing a lot of diet stories, but when you're thrown into a medical eating issue like that, you're just like, 'All the things I was told about food and bodies don't apply here.' That's when I started to see how much anxiety about controlling my body has really backfired for me. Like, if I was going to try to make eating seem like a fun, great thing to do for my kid, maybe I needed to stop being afraid of bread."

Even parents like Sole-Smith, who are vocal and persistent in their goal to raise kids with minimal interference from diet culture, often find their attempts thwarted by a fatphobic society that fails to take into account the very real damage that even "well-intended" weight-shaming can do to a child's developing psyche. In January 2023, the American Academy of Pediatrics released a set of guidelines for evaluating and treating children and young adults with obesity that controversially advised health-care providers to refer children as young as two to "intensive health behavior and lifestyle treatment" programs for a too-high BMI. Sole-Smith expressed her worry about the guidelines in a *New York Times* op-ed, writing: "We cannot solve anti-fat bias by making fat kids thin. Our current approach only teaches them that trusted adults believe the bullies are right—that a fat body is just a problem to solve. That's not where the conversation about anyone's health should begin."

It's not just the medical establishment that Sole-Smith sees as culpable for the increasing pressure on kids to avoid gaining excess weight at any cost, though; all too often, that pressure can be applied by parents themselves. While other parents often come to Sole-Smith with desperate questions about how to inculcate positive body image and a love of food in their kids, they're rarely ready to accept the possibility of fatness in their families as anything other than a long-shadowed boogeyman. "These parents want to ensure that their kids don't have eating disorders, but they also want to ensure thinness, and you can't really have it both ways," says Sole-Smith. It's always painful for me to watch parents restrict their children's eating and/or criticize their bodies—whether it's on TV or in real life, on the playground while I babysit—but I can't help feeling some empathy, too; I know how hard it can be to commence the internal work of placing physical health and mental well-being above smallness, whether it's for yourself or even for your child.

The COVID-19 pandemic has only underscored how badly America's mothers are suffering without the sort of societal safety net that is provided by subsidized child care in Finland,

South Korea, Denmark, and other countries. According to an American Psychological Association study published in March 2021, about 42 percent of US adults gained weight—twenty-nine pounds, on average—since the start of the pandemic. Plenty of articles have been written about coming to terms with, and embracing, that pandemic weight, but I still can't help thinking about those new pounds accumulating on the bodies of mothers across the country, mothers who are already maxed out and, in many cases, ill prepared to add the task of "modeling positive attitudes toward weight fluctuations" for their children. How many children will grow up in the shadow of the "quarantine fifteen," learning that weight gain is inherently bad (even if it comes during an unprecedented global pandemic and enforced period of isolation)?

My mother once told me that her biggest fear was losing me, but if she ever did, she had a plan. She would drive out to the middle of the country—somewhere she didn't know anyone—rent a cheap apartment, and eat and drink herself to death. She was joking, of course, one hand wrapped around a wineglass and the other affectionately patting my head, but I thought about the scenario from time to time, only with myself in the driver's seat, the cheap apartment. I pictured myself sitting in a chair in a nondescript room, surrounded by crinkly chip bags and extra-large tubs of ice cream, window shades down, nobody around for miles. It was awful, I knew, just an awful way to think, but I indulged myself nonetheless. I thought of that sickening fantasy again when I read *The Recovering*, Leslie Jamison's stirring 2018 account of a life marked by alcoholism and anorexia, and there came across a Raymond

Carver poem I'd never bothered to slog through firsthand when he'd been assigned in any number of my English classes. Titled "Luck," the poem describes a child making his way through the aftermath of his parents' debauched party, ending with the stanza:

> *Years later,*
> *I still wanted to give up*
> *friends, love, starry skies,*
> *for a house where no one*
> *was home, no one coming back,*
> *and all I could drink.*

The genius of "Luck" lies in Carver's ability to zero in on the mental gymnastics that those of us who struggle with addiction—to alcohol, drugs, food, or any other vice—are so skilled at performing. "I'll trade this for that," we tell ourselves, shutting out friends and family alike in favor of the seductive pull of solitude and the freedom it brings—freedom to stop pretending, to let our masks slip, to indulge ourselves in a momentary reprieve from judgment. I can't count how many times I've canceled plans or "gone to bed early" in order to be alone with food over the past twenty-nine years; I'd be even less capable of counting how many times I've wanted to. Throughout my life, my mother has filled her kitchen with life, laughter, and food, even if it was of the skinless-chicken-breast-and-salad variety; why, then, was my greatest dream as a child to be completely alone in that same kitchen with the lights off and the fridge stocked, sucking colored frosting from the tube with abandon and chasing it with tasteless mouthfuls of soft, pliant white bread?

When I began to gain "real" weight (as in, more than a few pounds) during the early quarantine phase of the COVID-19 pandemic, the hardest part wasn't making my peace with my brand-new stretch marks, or dipping into my rapidly dwindling savings for larger clothes that actually fit, or even the slow, sometimes-agonizing process of learning to treat my new body with care; it was the imagined threat of my mother's disapproval. Learning to acclimate my mom and Flavia to my relatively new, hard-won policy of *no dieting and no diet talk* has taken some work, but from an adult perspective, the idea that my issues with food are all somehow my mother's fault seems to fall along the too-familiar lines of "Hey, when all else fails, blame women!" Did anyone support my mom—or any of our mothers—in developing a relationship with food and with her body that wasn't toxic? If not, could they have been expected to perfectly support us? The good news is, it takes only one mother actively working on her relationship with food and body image—and one daughter watching, listening, and quietly learning—to begin to disrupt the cycle, paving the way for at least the possibility of hard-won body peace.

Chapter 2

FEAR

There's a lot from my teenage years that I hope I'll someday forget—including, but not limited to, the proper procedure for shotgunning a Mike's Hard Lemonade and the time I accidentally dropped my prescription deodorant in the middle of my ninth-grade English classroom for everyone to see—but the item highest on my laundry list of "Emma's Would-Be Repressed Memories" is the sight of Keira Knightley's hip bones emerging proudly from the expanse between a pubic bone–grazing pair of jeans and a halter top fashioned entirely from sequins. They were canyons, deep and seemingly infinite, as though within their shallows they might be able to hold all the mysteries of the world.

If you, like me, watched the 2002 rom-com *Bend It Like Beckham* on a loop throughout the early aughts, you're probably all too familiar with Knightley in this outfit. In the movie, she plays Jules, an *extremely* dyke-coded soccer star who can normally be found breaking her mother's heart with her penchant for sports bras and track shorts, thus making Jules's sequined sartorial glow-up for an evening out at a German nightclub all the more impressive. Jules doesn't get the guy at the end of the movie, but to my warped teen mind, she got a bigger prize: she got to be thin, bony-elbowed, knobby-hipped, and impossibly graceful in spite of it all. I know now that it's ridiculous to project bodily perfection onto anyone, celebrity or no, but when I was fourteen, sitting spellbound in front of my best friend Jazmine's family room TV on yet another Saturday night when nobody from our high school had invited us out, being Keira Knightley in *Bend It Like Beckham*—beautiful, sporty, so slender I wanted to cast off any evidence of my own body when confronted with the perceived perfection of hers—seemed like simultaneously the safest and most exciting thing a young woman could be.

I was big into bodily camouflage that year, constantly on alert for ways my physical form could betray me. The aforementioned prescription deodorant I'd ordered online was applied in stealth, in the seldom-used girls' locker room on the ground floor of the school gym. I owned two identical lace-trimmed camis, the kind it seemed like the government more or less issued to American girls who'd been born between 1990 and 1995, and I wore one of the two under a regular shirt every single day, stretching its hem all the way to the midthigh point of my jeans in an attempt to hide the hips that seemed to widen by the day. When I couldn't get away with that cami-optical illusion, I stuck to big-girl tradition and wrapped sweaters around my waist, hoping the effect was more "gotta get to the pep rally!" than "unpopular ninth grader trying to remain invisible." I was new that year, starting over after a miserable eighth-grade year marked primarily by the fact that approximately zero of the thirty-eight other girls in my class at my Upper East Side all-girls' prep school ("the one *Gossip Girl* was based on," I got used to telling people, waiting for their reaction) would deign to speak to me anymore.

I hadn't exactly been crushin' it socially 24/7 in the years since my family moved back to New York in 2001, but grades three through seven went smoothly enough for me, if you didn't count my parents splitting up when I was in fourth grade (amicably, it should be said, but that's not really the kind of perspective an eight-year-old brings to the situation) or the fact that I was always in danger of failing math and/or science. I always had at least one best friend to gossip and conspire with at any given time, and in sixth grade—the same year our school brought in a *Today Show* nutritionist to give us a lecture on the dangers of the "eat one ice cream sandwich and nothing else all day" diet that had been sweeping the cafeteria—I improbably found my way to the center of a clique of girls who were, if not the *coolest* in our grade (you needed Repetto ballet flats and understated yet clearly expensive Tiffany jewelry for that), at least objectively more cool-adjacent than any other group I'd belonged to before.

If you've ever seen a teen movie or had the misfortune of being or raising a thirteen-year-old girl, you probably know what happened next: they ditched me, either because I was a raging, unfixable, boy-repelling nerd (my interpretation at the time) or because teenage girls are generally not the most loyal bunch (my interpretation after a whole lot of therapy). Either way, I found myself alone a lot during my eighth-grade year, and food was always there to fill the friendship void. My house wasn't the kind that overflowed with snack food, but I soon learned to line the cabinets of my bedside table with marshmallows and Reese's Peanut Butter Cups from the CVS on Broadway or the bodega a block from my house, hoarding spoons from my mom's kitchen and eating in secret when she thought I was asleep; at my dad's place just one block over, I ate fancy La Perruche sugar cubes by the handful, standing up in the small tiled kitchen and grazing on my stash like a horse in its stable. I made a habit of searching the house for loose change, paying for my binge bounty in quarters and dimes.

One of my clearest binge memories from that time is so on-the-nose that I don't even like to think about it, much less describe it; even now, it feels less like a memory than a glimpse of a scene I saw on some treacly after-school special. It was the night of the annual Christmas party at an ultra-popular girl's house, an event so professionally catered and grand and well appointed, with icicle lights and fake ivy, that *everyone* in our grade (even marginal weirdos like myself) scored an invite. Things hadn't been good with my clique for a while, but I went—both to the popular girl's party and the preparty at preppy, square-featured Sarah's house before it, exchanging dollar-store gifts, doing my best to make everyone laugh—and for a while, things seemed fine. At some point, I learned that Sarah, Lydia, Lauren, and the rest of the friend group I'd prepartied with were planning a post-party sleepover, all six of them, sans me. A heartbreak, to be sure, but also a hallmark of middle school life for almost every girl, especially those of us who are marked with the label "different" for reasons we don't understand.

I can't remember how I got home from the popular girl's party—did I take a cab? Did I even know how to hail a cab then? Did someone drop me off?—but later that night I found myself sitting in front of a *Friends* rerun at home alone, still in the festive lace party dress I'd bought with my mom at some fusty, now-shuttered boutique on Amsterdam, letting the blue glow of the TV illuminate the sight of me eating freely from a bowl of chocolate-chip cookie dough I'd cheerfully made and stuck in the fridge earlier that week. Soon after the sleepover debacle, Lauren messaged me on AIM to coldly ask me to bring the heels I'd borrowed from her for a bat mitzvah to school and "just leave them in [her] locker." Just like that, my ostracism was complete.

Somewhere around the middle of eighth grade, my teachers must have informed my parents that I was spending all my time at school alone; I sure didn't do it, hell-bent as I was on convincing my parents that I was okay. Nothing to worry about here, no sirree; I was a regular, factory-issue teenage girl, with plenty of friends to prove it, and if I didn't have a boyfriend or a crush, or even know any guys my age socially, well . . . *I* wasn't the one who had decided I should go to an all girls' school. I'd cobbled together an idea of what an American teenager was from my parents' friends' kids and from the sitcoms I mainlined on weekends, and the ways in which I wasn't her—wasn't pretty, wasn't popular, wasn't sporty or do-goody or constantly sliding in after curfew—felt burned into my skin. I knew, without ever articulating it to myself or anyone else, that I was failing at the one job I'd been given. Unsurprisingly, my impression of a normal, happy eighth grader wasn't good enough to convince my parents for long, and they quickly made last-minute arrangements to get me out of that school, pulling me out of class to have me take standardized tests that the other girls who were "applying out" had completed months ago. (I treasured every stolen out-of-school moment, savoring the time away from my classmates almost as much as the Starbucks wraps we'd pick up after.)

Eventually, I started ninth grade at the notoriously intimidating, competitive private K–12 in the tony Riverdale neighborhood of the Bronx that my cousins Mickey and Tim—my mom's oldest brother's kids, who lived in the same building as my mom and I did and who were more like my mean, funny, fart-joke-cracking older brothers than anything else—had attended, and while the intensity of the workload was stressed to me multiple times, it was clear to me from the start it would be more than just an academic challenge for me. When my mom borrowed my uncle's car to take me to freshman orientation at a 320-acre "nature lab" in Connecticut, either Mickey or Tim (or both of them) had left a note in the glove compartment reading "Tell Emma not to screw this weekend up; orientation is huge for her."

Screw it up I did, in a manner of speaking. I didn't make any inroads with my overwhelmingly blond, preternaturally cool classmates, most of whom had been carpooling to school together (some in parental SUVs, some in literal black cars) since they were four. I'd chosen my clothes with care, desperate to seem chill and put together, yet still somehow managed to appear for Day One of the weekend's outdoorsy festivities in a purple-and-blue-striped rugby shirt identical to the one worn by a quiet math nerd who would later be expelled for stalking one of the popular girls I'd failed to ingratiate myself with that weekend. Plus, I was bad at any and all outdoor games, couldn't do trust falls, and was too scared to make eye contact with any boys.

I didn't exactly take my new school by storm on that nature lab trip, but I did meet the person who would quickly become my best friend, and—fifteen years later—remains one of the most important people in my life.

Jazmine was shorter than me by a few inches, with a mane of curly brown hair, thoughtful green eyes, a slightly upturned nose, and a closet full of the kind of three-quarter-length-sleeve cashmere cardigans and Tory Burch ballet flats I knew I needed to get my hands on if I wanted to fit in (it would take months before I learned that almost anything nice Jazmine wore, she'd stolen from her young, cool mom's closet). We'd both moved to New York at eight—her from London, Ontario, me from Rome, Italy—and we were both quiet, bookish children of divorce with a penchant for sketch comedy and browsing around Urban Outfitters for hours, pulling one another in for fitting room consults on an ironic T-shirt or an ugly peplum as though we were actually ever going to buy anything.

If Jazmine's and my friendship didn't begin with food, it was certainly anchored by it. After school, we'd take the 1 train to Chipotle for burritos the size of newborn babies or to Peaches for aggressively average frozen yogurt or, occasionally, the A/C/E all the way to Queens for the Indian buffet at Jackson Diner, studying for art history exams and reciting our favorite '90s-era *Saturday Night Live* punch lines and cackling away over inscrutable inside jokes made at our classmates' expense. (There was one girl we referred to solely as "Fast-Talking High Trousers" for four years, due to her propensity for tight jeans and hurried speech. In retrospect, we may not have been nice girls.)

Throughout high school, Jazmine was my ballast, and even though nobody else at school spoke to us, we kept up a semi-convincing front of not caring; who needed football games and first dates and parties in someone's parent-free Park Avenue apartment when we had well-worn VHS tapes of every aughts rom-com ever made to rewatch, Saturday night after Saturday night for four years straight, in Jazmine's basement?

In retrospect, I'm grateful that we managed to eke out a relatively wholesome New York City adolescence when a not-insignificant number of our classmates were already living more-or-less adult lives straight out of *Succession*, but at the time, my eighth-grade *Heathers* experience loomed large, and—unwilling to trust my social instincts, knowing they'd somehow failed me before without my noticing—I used Jazmine as my compass for everything, food included. If she had a cafeteria turkey sandwich for lunch, I had one, too; if she managed to resist the Duncan Hines boxed brownie mix sitting in the kitchen pantry on yet another weekend night in, I did, too (and conversely, if she got dessert, I did, too, already learning to base my food "yeses" and "nos" on what I thought was acceptable, not what I wanted).

The wild thing is, like so many teenage girls, I *wasn't actually fat* in high school. I'd been a skinny kid who'd packed on pubescent weight like so much bubble-wrap padding, but once it settled, I was probably never more than ten pounds overweight. Still, I felt each pound hanging from my bones like an indictment, sure that if I could just be skinny enough to wear shorts to school without worrying about how my thighs splayed out on my chair in class, everything else in my life would fall into place. High school was the first, but not the last, time I used my body as a proxy for everything I couldn't name and couldn't fix; when I look back at the few teen photos of me that have survived on Facebook (the aughts digital equivalent of the shoebox full of photos under the bed, recording you forever in the physical incarnations you might have preferred to forget), I see a girl crying out to be noticed, to be liked, to be pulled into someone else's story, and I thought all those things could happen only if I was thin.

According to the National Center on Addiction and Substance Abuse, 62.3 percent of American teenage girls report actively trying to lose weight, a number that surprises me only because it isn't higher. After all, we live in the era of waist trainers and "Ozempic face," Instagram weight-loss ads and dramatic Kardashian slim downs; I didn't think pop culture could get much more thinness-obsessed than it was when I was coming of age, but the era of social media has proved me wrong once again. Yes, today's teenagers have fat icons like Paloma

Elsesser and Barbie Ferreira and Aidy Bryant to look up to, but representation can go only so far, or do so much. At a certain point, when we're still selling diet plans to kids and rewarding grown women for fitting into sample sizes, I think we have to admit that our national obsession with being small isn't just some tragic holdover from the aughts; its affirmation of white supremacist, cis-heteropatriarchal notions about physical appearance and intrinsic worth—which Sabrina Strings expertly unpacks in her 2019 book *Fearing the Black Body*, detailing "the history and legacy of the preference for slimness and aversion to fatness, with attention to their racial, gender, class, and medical contours"—is a tricky shape-shifter, finding its way into cultural narratives where it shouldn't belong just as we proudly tell ourselves we've exorcized it forever.

Throughout my own adolescence, fat was the third rail; it was the thing I was taught to pity and disdain, the one thing I knew I couldn't be if I wanted to be loved. And really, is there anything we've taught teenage girls to crave more than any scrap of love they can get their hands on? Maybe that's why, when I learned that the Ritalin a kindly adolescent psychiatrist had prescribed in hopes of getting my grades up also functioned as an appetite suppressant, I was thrilled; it seemed like a magical cure, something straight out of a fairy tale. To just . . . *not be hungry*, all of a sudden, to not be pulled toward the siren call of food, all because of a pill I'd taken?

Appetite loss wasn't the only Ritalin side effect I was chasing. I also liked the way the pale-green pills seemed to make sleep optional, leaving me awake all night to study my French vocab flash cards and work away at the chemistry equations that stymied me during daylight hours. My grades soon improved, if marginally, and I now like to joke that my high school taught me a valuable lesson: there are twenty-four hours in any given day in which to work, so long as you have the right meds. I was hardly the only student popping pills at school, but the other kids seemed to take them to excel; I took them just to break even, and to calm the gnawing hunger beneath my ribs that it seemed like I'd been born with.

It's possible that a lower dose of Ritalin would have made more sense for me, or at least wouldn't have kept me up counting the bathroom tiles until 3:00 a.m. on school nights, but I didn't know that my constant jumpiness and wakefulness and inability to eat wasn't normal, and my parents weren't the type to micromanage my habits or force-feed me (apart from the morning of the SATs, when my mom insisted I swallow a dish of blueberries "for brain food"; two hours later, I found myself anxiety-puking blue gunk in the bathroom). Plus, like so many teenage girls, especially those nursing budding eating disorders, I was secretive as hell, unwilling to let my parents in on the secret of the little green pills; they knew I was taking them, obviously, but they didn't know how ardently I willed that medication to erase me, to make my stomach flatten and my bones show.

In retrospect, knowing what I know now about the prevalence of teen eating disorders, I'm grateful I wasn't worse off. I experimented with throwing up my meals a few times in high school, but then—as now—found the whole bulimia thing to be uncomfortably physical. I ate—I *eat*—in order to temporarily anesthetize myself, to forget about my body, not to be confronted with its heaving, sweating limitations on my knees in front of a toilet. In sixth grade, I stole a copy of Steven Levenkron's 1979 novel *The Best Little Girl in the World* from the school library, marveling at the story of teen ballerina Francesca—or "Kessa," as she preferred to be called—and her downslide into severe anorexia.

The Best Little Girl in the World is, in a way, a perfect emblem of most mainstream eating-disorder narratives, focusing as it does on an upper-middle-class, white, New York City–dwelling, perfectionist female dancer who restricts her eating until she's below the eighty-pound mark. With the benefit of hindsight, I can see that I took away a lot of incorrect ideas about what an eating disorder was from that book; I was from the city, too, white and female, with parents who had enough money to pay for my medical treatment just like Kessa's did, but I thought that I, with my messy hair and room and bad grades, couldn't possibly have anything in common with hyper-neat, obsessive Kessa. On some level, I even bought into the book's wild supposition that only white, affluent women could suffer from eating disorders. (Lila, Kessa's Black roommate in the hospital she's sent to after losing too much weight, tells her: "You always had enough food, so you can make a game out of it. Maybe when blacks have enough they'll start makin' a game out of it too.")

Today, I can see how much preteen me shared with Kessa. I wasn't a full-blown binge eater yet, but I think I recognized something in Kessa's calorie counting, in her watchfulness and secrecy, and the shoved-down anger at her family she was able to confront only in treatment. What struck me most, though, was Kessa's fear and exhaustion; she fights her body at every turn, desperately denying its need for food and doing her best to dance or starve off every calorie, and by the time she manages to connect with a kindly therapist during her hospitalization, it's clear how long she's been suffering under the strain of trying to be the perfect daughter. (This is in contrast to her all-star brother, Gregg, and wild-child sister, Susannah, who command the lion's share of their parents' attention even when Kessa is hospitalized.)

Kessa's need to be perfect is a great burden, to be sure, but it's also a kind of privilege. Anorexia has been portrayed as a disease of privilege in countless schlocky TV movies and magazine features illustrated by photos of sad-eyed white girls in leotards staring at their ever-shrinking forms in the mirror, and despite the efforts of groups like the National Eating Disorder Association (NEDA), many people still aren't fully aware that the real disparity within anorexia appears not in incidence, but in diagnosis and cultural competence around care. This state of affairs wasn't confined to a 1970s-era understanding of eating disorders and racial identity either; as *Hood Feminism* author Mikki Kendall wrote in a *New York Times* essay in 2021: "The lingering cultural myth that eating disorders are the province of white women isn't just misleading: It also keeps us from addressing the uniquely insidious factors that can cause black women to hate their bodies."

The Best Little Girl in the World—written, as it was, in 1979— can't be expected to hold up today as an inclusive (or even accurate) depiction of real-world disordered eating, but when I reread it now, I'm bowled over by the quick mention the book makes of binge eating. "Bingeing is going all out," Kessa's bossy hospital hallmate Myrna, a fellow anorexic who also dabbles in bingeing and purging, tells her, adding, "You know, when you hit the fridge and eat your way straight through it in one sitting. I do it all the time. Before they put me in I was doing it every day. I'm probably the world's best binger." Was that the first reference to binge eating I ever encountered, back in sixth grade? Did it even flag anything to me, anorexic-in-training that I was at the time, or did I make sense of it only a few years later, once my friends ditched me and I began to spend Saturday nights telling my parents I was going to the gym and instead hunching on a bench in nearby Riverside Park with an economy-size bag of Candy Cane Hershey's Kisses?

As it turns out, I was far from the only person my age who spent their teen years learning to skip meals and count calories and find unassailable perfection in Keira Knightley's hip bones. Sabrina Imbler, currently a staff writer at the sports and culture website *Defector* and the author of the 2022 essay collection *How Far the Light Reaches: A Life in Ten Sea Creatures*, spent their teen years in San Francisco's Bay Area worshiping at the altar of Knightley-esque physical proportions, though they were less preoccupied by *Bend It Like Beckham* than by Knightley's period roles in movies like *Atonement* and *Pride and Prejudice*. "I remember wishing so badly that I could look like her," Imbler says of Knightley, adding that in addition to mega-famous celebrities, they also obsessed at length over the looks of female friends and classmates.

"I think a lot of that was wrapped up in me not understanding that I was queer," says Imbler, adding, "I was looking at these people's bodies and desiring so much and not really getting how much of that was *Do I want to look like this person or do I want to be with this person?*" Like me, Imbler didn't come out as queer until their early twenties, but queer or not, when you've presented as and been socialized as a female in post-aughts American society, it can be hard to shed the feeling that another person's body—even the body of someone you love and crave and trust completely—exists as a kind of reproach to your own.

Imbler describes the experience of learning to diet as a teen from their mother, who immigrated to Michigan from Taiwan as a teen, in their book, writing: "She wanted me to be white so things would be easier. Skinny, so things would be easier. Straight, so things would be easy, easy, easy. So that, unlike her, no one would ever question my right to be here, in America." Imbler also knows the specific experience of growing up perennially on the social outs in a hyper-wealthy environment, telling me: "Popularity hierarchy at my school was very much sorted with thinness and whiteness at the top. I grew up thinking that because I went to school with kids like the son of Steve Jobs, who were all thin and white, that it really affected my understanding of my own family's affluence."

I, too, never thought of myself as "rich" in high school, even though my family undoubtedly was by most of the country's standards; within the funhouse-mirror world of New York private school, though, having two journalist parents who both lived on the Upper West Side and had enough money to pay my full tuition barely distinguished me among the sea of very rich, mostly white kids I was being educated alongside. (In fact, sometimes even my objectively cushy background had earned me ignorant comments; I still remember one button-nosed blond girl asking me after play practice in sixth grade if we had movie theaters on the Upper West Side, which today just makes me shudder to imagine what kind of questions she and her friends were posing to the few girls in our class who commuted from Brooklyn or Harlem.)

In retrospect, being surrounded by so much privilege was a convenient way of avoiding accountability for the not-small share of it that I myself possessed, but at the time, I genuinely thought that Jazmine and I were weird for doing nothing more with our time than hitting up Subway with the $10 our parents would slip us now and then, and the girls whose parents spent thousands to keep them in Juicy Couture sweats and to send them to all manner of high-achieving summer "enrichment camps" were the normal ones. None of those girls ever seemed to eat much in the cafeteria, and on my few academics-related excursions to their houses, I saw that it ran in the family; their moms favored Carr's Table Water Crackers and celery and any other crunchy, low-calorie, distinctly WASPy snack, hiding—or, more likely, instructing the housekeeper to hide—the telltale green bag of Tate's Chocolate-Chip Cookies behind the shelves' worth of steel-cut oatmeal and low-carb cereal.

Eating disorders were long understood—erroneously, of course—as a disease of affluence, with a doctor in *The Best Little Girl in the World* reassuring Kessa's frightened parents that "we do know it affects girls from good homes, upper and middle class." This logic has now been thoroughly debunked by the medical community, with a 2021 study in the peer-reviewed scientific journal *Eating Behaviors* concluding that "there is no pattern of evidence for a relationship between higher socioeconomic status and eating disorders; eating disorders present across a wide range of socioeconomic backgrounds." When you're a weird, marginal kid trying to blend into a hyper-competitive, affluent early-aughts environment, though, thinness can be the quickest route to the kind of self-alteration I think every lonely nerd dreams of at one time or another.

I don't remember more than a handful of fat students attending my high school, and it probably goes without saying that the popular kids—the ones who played on the sports teams, led the student-run clubs, made everyone laugh with cheeky announcements at assemblies—were almost always thin. Thinness seemed less like a virtue on its own than a shortcut by which I might be able to access their ease in their bodies, their apparent comfort with being noticed. (When I first read the novel *Prep* in tenth grade, I noted protagonist Lee Fiora's silent, watchful way of tracking the habits of cooler, wealthier classmates at her intimidating East Coast boarding school and thought: *There I am.*)

Of course, I know now that merely being thin doesn't mean you're not wrestling with weight and body issues (I, after all, was technically within the healthy weight range for my height during high school), but with the solipsism so common among teenagers, I convinced myself I was the only one struggling; when I looked at other girls' bodies, all I felt—or, to Imbler's point about desire and repressed queerness, all I allowed myself to feel at the time—was envy of their fearlessness in scanty tops and denim short-shorts. To be popular, I told myself, was to never feel jiggly or flabby or unwanted or alone; aloneness, or near-aloneness, had been my habitual social state for long enough by then that I couldn't imagine anything I desired more.

"At my school, there was the popular circle and the un-popular circle, and the second one was definitely my circle," re-calls Imbler, noting that even floating beneath the cool-kid fray didn't protect them from wanting to be thin; in fact, it may have stoked their passion to lose weight, encouraging them to seek out relationships that mirrored how they felt about their body. "I remember I had one friend, who was also Asian, and we were very honest with each other about our hatred for our bodies and our desire to look like other people. I think we both knew we couldn't bring that stuff to our other friends, but we believed something to be genuinely wrong and bad about ourselves," says Imbler.

Teenagers so often bond over wrongness, real or perceived, and while movies like *Ghost World* and *Whip It* tend to depict nerdy friend pairs as model-beautiful girls (in glasses and bad clothes, of course) who are too enthralled with each other to even notice how ostracized they are, I know Jazmine and I both secretly worried about how unpopular—not even unpopular, *unknown*—we were, particularly at the beginning of high school, before we'd gained the requisite feminist-blogosphere-enabled snarkiness necessary to dismiss the popular kids as boring fu-ture tech bros unworthy of our attention. The anxiety I'd felt in eighth grade about my parents discovering just how friend-less and miserable I was never really left me during my teen years, mushrooming instead into a larger terror of them figuring out just how friendless and miserable Jazmine and I *both* were from ninth through twelfth grade. To be lonely was one thing, to know Jazmine was lonely, too, right alongside me, was another.

Jazmine and I retook the same stultifyingly boring dance class for PE credit every year, four years in a row, and while I've forgotten the choreography and blessedly put out of my mind the earth-toned leotards we had to wear, I still remember being pierced by one of the Harry Nilsson lyrics we danced to: "Two can be as bad as one / It's the loneliest number since the number one." Now, fifteen years and two fully fleshed-out personal lives later, I can't believe my friendship with Jazmine—the bride whose wedding I gave a toast at two summers ago, the gifted editor who's given notes on almost anything important I've ever published, the blue iChat bubble texting me as I write this—was ever a source of shame to me, but I know it was; not shame in anything about *her*, but shame at our mutual failure to thrive in our new environment coupled with a paralyzing, unspoken fear that life would always be like this.

Of course, bonding intensely with one friend—over bodies, over thinness, or just over the daily difficulty of existing in the world as a teenager—isn't an uncommon experience for young people across the gender spectrum. Writer Isle McElroy, whose novel *The Atmospherians* came out in 2021 and who has written about their history with bulimia in online essays like "The Prob-lem with the Stories We Tell About Eating Disorders," which was featured in *The Atlantic*, was less focused on possessing a celebrity's physique in high school—"I never really had any belief that that was something I could obtain," they recall—and more attuned to the bodies of the people around them.

"My grandmother constantly compared me to my cousins, who were always outside playing sports, and I was always being asked why I was in the house eating," says McElroy of growing up as an only child in rural New Jersey, recalling the body-centric relationship they had with a close friend at fifteen: "He decided that he would be my personal trainer, and as someone who lived close to me and was a year older, his body took on a lot of power for me. At the time when I was losing weight and my eating disorder was considered to be at its worst, I got obsessed with wearing his younger brother's soccer jersey and being part of his family; I wanted to become him, essentially."

In their 2018 *Tin House* essay "Hazardous Cravings," McElroy revisits their high school stint working at the local Dairy Queen, describing their journey into the minefield of ED culture; they binged, purged, and restricted their way through a significant weight loss, but were discomfited at how the world met them once they'd shed a certain number of pounds: "Dieting had been simple. It had given me rules, structured my life. As I lost weight, people supported me, but they owed me nothing now that I was skinny." (I can attest that is one of the weirdest things about losing weight, something our culture encourages us to do at every turn; as it turns out, some people are just more comfortable with fat people when we stay in the box marked "fat" that they've so generously apportioned out to us.)

In their *Tin House* essay, McElroy describes the envy they felt toward their friend and DQ coworker Boots's relationship with food, writing: "Boots ate with unselfconscious abandon, the way I had eaten in my early days, concocting with a mad scientist's frenzy, mixing hard ice cream with soft serve, marshmallow topping with cherries, mint syrup with Heath bits—flavor combinations be damned—just to test how it tasted." The writing is beautiful and the sentiment is painfully pure (who *wouldn't* want to eat like a confident teenage boy?), but when McElroy and I talk about it in the fall of 2022—a year after McElroy came out publicly as nonbinary and began using "they/them" pronouns—they're not sure they would express themselves today the way they had in *Tin House.*

"It's striking to me how repressed I was, and how there's this hole in the essay that would today read, '*Dieting gave me access to femininity in ways that I so desperately wanted,*'" says McElroy. "That relationship with Boots was really interesting to me, because there was love and affection there, but also competition, right? Reading the essay now is so interesting, because it almost feels like the way an anthropologist would talk about a country where they've only been once. Masculinity was sort of like, 'I don't want to be here, but I'm going to talk about it a lot.'"

It doesn't escape my notice that Imbler, McElroy, and I are all queer adults whose adolescent periods of disordered eating overlapped with our time in the closet. Obviously, members of the LGBTQ+ community don't have a monopoly on bodily dissatisfaction, but it makes sense that if you know on some level in high school that you're different (or, even if you won't admit it to yourself that you know, the people around you somehow seem to), you might focus even harder on shrinking yourself down or pumping yourself up or mastering the art of the midnight binge and purge or whatever else might distract the world from what's going on inside you. Unfortunately, the evidence seems to suggest that Imbler's, McElroy's, and my collective dissatisfaction with ourselves as teenagers was hardly a relic from the aughts: the Trevor Project announced a new research brief in 2022 that found that LGBTQ+ youth experience eating disorders at higher rates than their cishet peers, also noting that eating disorders are underdiagnosed in LGBTQ+ youth because medical professionals often fail to detect and name the symptoms.

There's something comforting about talking to people who share a base-level understanding, not only of who you are today, but of who you were years ago, overflowing with self-imposed hunger and too scared of the world beyond Weight Watchers—or any other spartan diet regime—to allow yourself to take up space. Engaging with Imbler and McElroy about the eating disorders (full-blown or putative) that characterized our teen years is calming to the part of my brain that still secretly worries I'm the only one like this, in spite of the evidence that at least 9 percent of the US population will have an eating disorder in their lifetime, but it's also sad in a way I can't quite explain.

In the back of my mind, I picture the three of us, each fanned out in our separate school cafeterias across the United States over the span of a decade, counting calories and avoiding dessert and despairing over the physical forms that—at the very moment that we lamented them—would never be younger.

Next, I picture kids all over the country and the world, kids in classrooms and locker rooms and on soccer fields and in 4H meetings, kids who come from all variety of zip codes and racial and ethnic and socioeconomic backgrounds yet somehow all seem to know nothing so fiercely and fully as they know that their own bodies are wrong; not just the Kessas of the world, but all the kids whose eating disorders aren't caught or treated, all the ones silently suffering from a profound lack of internalized self-regard.

It's hard to picture, but I'm glad that at least Imbler and McElroy and I and the many other LGBTQ+ people I know who have struggled with disordered eating are starting to talk about it, to write about it, to turn our problems over to one another and to therapists and to the general custody of the world around us. God knows, we've let fear run us—and our relationships with our bodies—long enough.

Chapter 3

LOSE

In 2010, news broke that the actress Ginnifer Goodwin—known primarily for playing affable, "best friend"–adjacent characters in movies like *Mona Lisa Smile* and *Win a Date with Tad Hamilton!*— had been on Weight Watchers since she was nine. The backlash was swift, with many questioning the decision-making of parents who would subject their children to diet culture so early in life. I was sixteen then, reading the exclamation-point-heavy Jezebel comments on my laptop before school, experiencing a strange mix of gratification at their outrage and smugness at my own superior sense of agency. After all, I'd been *twelve* when I'd started Weight Watchers, and the idea to join had been entirely my own, the monthly dues paid for with babysitting money; I had nobody to blame, and nobody to thank.

I kept paying for Weight Watchers on and off throughout the first year of high school, then abandoned it altogether until midway through my senior year of college at a small liberal arts school in the middle of Ohio, when I stepped on a scale for the first time after a junior year spent in Russia subsisting exclusively on pelmeni and marked-up Starbucks holiday lattes and didn't like what I saw. I'd spent my late teens and early twenties trying out keto, gluten-free, and a host of other "eating plans" by then, but Weight Watchers was a kind of return to childhood, a sad little homecoming. I still knew the system by heart, knew what various foods corresponded to what point values (five points for half an avocado, four for a glass of wine, bananas are free!); mostly, though, I knew that Weight Watchers had been there for me before, a desperately needed—if leaky—life raft in a churning sea of body anxiety and self-hatred.

For a while, things were okay. I logged my meals dutifully, recording each cup of dining hall fro-yo and late-night stoned handful of tortilla chips until they gradually grew fewer. I started swimming laps in the Olympic-size campus pool I'd previously barely registered the existence of, having written off anything that took place in the school's capacious gym as "jock shit." I remember washing dishes in my campus apartment one afternoon between classes and noting idly that it had been a while since I'd trundled to the market in town for a pint of sorrow-drowning Ben & Jerry's; I would think about this moment later, recalling the days when I merely noticed what I was or wasn't eating without the hot rush of ensuing judgment. I lost ten pounds, then twenty, then thirty, then forty; by the time graduation rolled around, I was lighter than I'd been since ninth grade.

Later, when things turned, I longed for so much from my

college days; not just the glow that lit me up from within when a classmate complimented my weight loss, but the immediacy with which it began to pay off. After a college career spent solo while my friends coupled up, hookups suddenly became available to me (or maybe they always had been; maybe the problem was my confidence, not my body, but I wasn't ready to see that yet—I'm not sure I'm even ready now). I hooked up with two guys in two weeks toward the end of senior year, first a sunny blond frat bro who had a penchant for pairing pink polo shirts with purple knee-length shorts, then a sweet, dark-haired art major who referred to me by my full name—Emma Specter—like I was a girl he'd thought about. The sex was okay, I guessed, but what I really liked was seeing my body through their eyes; the hollows of my stomach, the knobby delicacy of my collarbone. I still felt a sick shame in the pit of my stomach in the morning when they left, but it was less like an overpowering stomach flu, more like a mild bug.

As much weight as I lost that year, I managed to keep some semblance of my sanity. After graduation, a group of friends and I took a trip to Rehoboth Beach, and I managed to put Weight Watchers on pause for the week, cracking crabs and devouring lobster rolls and downing sugary margaritas that always held the faint aftertaste of chlorine. I was so happy that week in my two-piece bathing suit, lying in the sun with my best friends and eating what I wanted when I wanted—or, at least, that's how I came to remember it. I don't know if there was a time in my adolescent or adult life that was totally untouched by my eating disorder, but until my mid-twenties, I moved in and out of a state that looked, in retrospect, something like peace—if not with my body, then at least with food.

I can't pinpoint exactly when things slipped out of my control, when dieting turned from one part of my life to its sum total. That's precisely the problem for so many disordered eaters who force ourselves to live by the rules of the diet industry; the goalposts in our heads keep moving without our consent, turning what was once a target weight into a prime example of what we swear we'll never be again. (Because, of course, to the disordered eater's mind, weight is not something we carry, it's something we *are*.) At some point after college, I know I put a pause on my Weight Watchers membership; was it that summer, a summer when I lived at home and drank a lot, took pills from the unlabeled bowl in my friends' minuscule East Village apartment, and went home with guys I wouldn't recognize in daylight? It makes sense that I would have lapsed in self-regulation at that time, a time when the question of who I was and who I would be loomed so large in my mind that I could barely breathe; I'd found new, inventive, decidedly "adult" ways to hate myself, so food was briefly allowed to recede into the background while I experimented with sex and drugs and—well, not rock 'n' roll, but a whole lot of whiny indie rock.

I moved to Los Angeles with my college friend Eliza in the fall of the year I graduated from college, and all I have from that time are mental snapshots. Me, biking eight miles a day from West Adams to Fairfax to report for my job as a web-series intern because I didn't have a car. Me, trying on size twenty-five jeans in a cramped Crossroads dressing room and noting with barely suppressed glee that they were too big, then remembering I still couldn't afford them. Me, alternately lonely and exhilarated in a city where I knew almost nobody. Me, skipping lunch and dinner, then sitting alone in a darkened office and bingeing on the stale leftover bagels and boxes of Trader Joe's candy that the writers hadn't finished during the workday, resolving to start fresh on Weight Watchers the next morning. Me, running my hands over my newly prominent hip bones in the solitude of my bed at night, conjuring some not-yet-existent boyfriend murmuring "You're too thin" and flushing with the imagined pleasure of it. In my mind, love was worshipful yet unobtrusive; I wanted someone to worry about me, but not to actually stop me from getting thinner.

Somewhere in the deepest recesses of Facebook there exist photos of me hiking in Death Valley with Eliza, raising my arms triumphantly over my head as we summit a hill, my sports-bra-clad torso pale and concave and—by almost anyone's account—small. I look happy in the photos, lean and confident; what I remember, though, is the oppressive heat that nearly bent me in two, the thirst that left my mouth agape, and, most of all, the hunger that gnawed at my insides with each step. I felt faint halfway through the eight-mile hike, but I didn't want to be dramatic about it (how many physical ailments have women ignored in the name of not being "dramatic"?), so I kept going. After the hike, we went to a steakhouse with a salad bar, and I distinctly remember feeling triumphant that I'd earned myself a generous pour of full-fat dressing. The calculus was so simple then: calories in, calories out. A day of hiking or biking or running plus a few skipped meals equaled the license to sit in the tub shoving semisweet chocolate chips into my mouth by the handful, tasting nothing, feeling nothing.

In the *Lifetime* movie of my life, these moments—getting dizzy in the Death Valley heat, bingeing in the bathtub—would have been artfully scored to communicate to the audience that Something Was Very Wrong. A friend or mentor would have intervened, I would have cried, a kind-eyed nutritionist would have been summoned, and a montage would show me going on long walks, cooking balanced meals, slowly getting better. In real life, nobody knew. Why would they? If my roommate Jenna—with whom I shared a semi-squalid one-bedroom in which we erected a complicated living room sheet tent to give her the illusion of privacy—ever noticed that the chocolate chips and peanut butter and Ritz crackers disappeared overnight from time to time, she never said anything. I was thin, but not scarily so, not enough to raise eyebrows (especially in the slenderness-obsessed City of Angels) or make my parents worry when they visited. Things *looked* fine, so I told myself they were.

There were so many things I desperately wanted in that strange, blurry expanse of LA time—professional success, a driver's license, a nicer apartment, a wide group of friends to go to dinner with in Silverlake and get drunk with in Frogtown—but I can't think of anything that pulled at me more than my desire for a boyfriend. I was thin, finally, and according to the rules of worth I'd established for myself long ago, that meant I was ready to love and be loved; so why didn't it ever work? Why did my sexual and (very occasionally) romantic encounters with men leave me restless, insatiable, hungry for care?

In her 2020 book *This Is Big: How the Founder of Weight Watchers Changed the World—and Me*, journalist and author Marisa Meltzer writes of the rich, abundant life that dieting promised her—and, poignantly, of all the ways in which it ultimately let her down. (This is perhaps the most insidious thing about diet culture: we're encouraged to think in terms of how we've failed at dieting, rather than examining the ways in which dieting has failed us.) Like me, Meltzer began dieting as a child, though she was five, not twelve, and her parents orchestrated her earliest attempts. Also like me, Meltzer went on and off Weight Watchers and other diets as an adult, striving for control of a body that had been a source of shame her whole life.

Meltzer is brutally honest about the ways in which her weight—or her feelings about her weight—have held her back in relationships, writing, "I blame everything that doesn't go well in my life, like dating, on my weight." To some degree, this one's on society; after all, 71 percent of plus-size women say they've been fat-shamed on standard dating apps, and as Charlotte Zoller wrote in a September 2020 installment of her *Teen Vogue* column "Ask a Fat Girl," many of us have earned our mistrust of dating while fat: "As fat women, we've learned to protect ourselves from the inevitable emotional pain associated with putting ourselves out there." It's so much easier to take yourself out of the running entirely, insisting you'll put together that Tinder profile in ten or twenty pounds, than it is to put yourself out into the world as an unabashed fat woman looking for love and deal with the world's often-exceptional cruelty.

One particularly complex aspect of fatness, though, is what

I like to call "fat exceptionalism"; media and diet culture would have us believe that our fat bodies are the exception, that anyone who loves them—and, thus, loves us—would have to be a rare gem who appreciates *what's on the inside*, even when 68 percent of American women are a size fourteen or above. We're firmly in the majority, yet that's cold comfort when you work in an industry that continues to prize thinness above all, as Meltzer and I do, or when you walk into a crowded Brooklyn bar for a first date and note that every other person there looks straight out of an Instagram ad for flat-tummy tea.

To enter the dating pool is, on some level, to put faith in the idea that you're worthy of love, or at least some hopefully good sex; to be fat is to be fed the insidious message at every turn that no, in fact, you are not. Is it any wonder that so many of us come back to diet culture again and again, despite knowing it rarely works in the long term? Diet culture is the mirage that turns desert sand into the appearance of life-giving water, the shimmering promise that if we just *committed*—just cut out carbs, just upped our treadmill routine, just tried a little harder—we'd have all the love and sex and fulfillment we could dream of. This is, of course, total bullshit; as Eliza once reminded me over sushi during yet another of my single-girl laments, "Being thin doesn't make you ready for a relationship. Everyone has their shit." I wish I'd listened to her then, instead of persisting in blaming every romantic downturn on my body (which, at the time, was barely heavy enough to menstruate regularly, but as it turns out, a lifelong fear of fat doesn't evaporate just because you've temporarily starved yourself down to a sample size). Oh, the things we force our bodies to bear when our minds aren't ready to carry the weight.

On its website, Weight Watchers boasts a full-on guide to "dating while losing weight" that includes tips like snacking before dinner so as not to get "hangry" (the horror!), sharing your entree (did you know one meal divided by two equals less points?), and when to let your date in on the dirty little secret that you are a living mammal engaged in the age-old practice of dieting. ("Remember: being honest about what makes you, you, makes you even more attractive.") If it sounds like I'm unfairly picking on Weight Watchers, I probably am; they are, after all, a business, and they stand to profit when you lose weight. (Actually, they stand to profit when you continually gain and lose the same ten pounds, but I digress.) It's in their best interest for you to slot everything else in your life—romance, friendship, work, family—around your diet; the real question is, is it in yours?

What frustrates me about the Weight Watchers dating guide is not its existence or the "advice" it dispenses, it's the fact that throughout my LA years, every word of it applied to me. I *did* eat before dates, to avoid ravenously gobbling up a distinctly unsexy plate of wings or fries; I *did* panic about how to make two glasses of wine last long enough to actually get to know someone, always doing the frantic mental math about whether one more round was worth a potential drunk binge that would lead to me waking up thick-tongued, puffy-eyed, and full of shame. My primary relationship in that stretch of time was with a menu, not whoever was on the other side of a bar table from me—I was, to put it simply, scared of men, so I worked even harder to be someone thin, someone they'd never leave, someone who could have her pick.

Now that we're almost three full years into the COVID-19 pandemic, old anxieties about "getting out there" are coming back in a big way. Meltzer says the best advice she got for dating while fat came from Megababe founder and plus-size influencer Katie Sturino: "Just show your body." It sounds easy, and for thin people, it very well might be; if you post accurate photos of your fat body, though, you're at far higher risk for rejection. "I can't believe it took me so long to wrap my head around the idea of just showing my body," says Meltzer. "People use filters and Facetune and all of that, and I certainly wasn't doing that, but I definitely wasn't showing my body off. I posted, you know, a few flattering selfies or whatever. And Katie was like, 'No, it should be: body shot, headshot, body shot, headshot.' It makes me so scared, but she's probably right; then you aren't hiding anything. There's this photographer who took Katie's super-hot online dating photos, so I hired him for a non-crazy amount of money, put on a couple of outfits I liked, and it was like, 'Yeah, that's my body. I'm not trying to obscure it. You make your own deduction.'"

Obscuring my body was a specialty of mine during my first forays into online dating, and for years, I kept specific photos high in the rotation; me on Halloween, dressed as Rabbi Raquel from *Transparent* in a long dress and tallit, the niche pop-culture reference and nod to my cultural Judaism less important to me than the definition of my jawline and the carved quality of my cheekbones. Me in a barely there cocktail dress at a dance party in Echo Park, the four-drinks-in dullness of my eyes trumped by the visible sinew of my arms and the concavity of my exposed thighs. Me in my sports bra in Death Valley, half starved and smiling. I told myself these photos showed I was fun, outdoorsy, a TV nut, but really, they showed I was skinny, encasing me forever at my post–Weight Watchers thinnest like a bug in amber.

My weight didn't actually fluctuate that much in my LA years—all that would come later, when I moved back to New York—but I lived in fear of every extra pound anyway, convinced that the contrast between my Tinder photos and the living reality of me shuffling into the bar in my clogs and cardigan would be too glaring for any date. Ironically, it was usually me who found reasons to reject the guys I went out with—this one was too sweaty, that one too boring, that other one too obsessed with Bitcoin—and even when a date did go well, I was less transfixed with the guy than with the potential for personal reinvention that he represented. I once went on a few dates with a moderately successful, significantly older TV writer who lived in a charming bungalow in Los Feliz; when I took a shower at his place the morning after we spent the night together for the first and only time, I was bowled over by the discovery that he had a *full set of guest towels*. (It doesn't take much to impress a twenty-three-year-old girl who's never had a boyfriend.)

The TV writer was everything I thought I wanted in a boyfriend—tall, Jewish, curly-haired, sardonic, employed—and when he ghosted me after our one and only sleepover, I was despondent. There's a particular kind of heartbreak to losing someone you didn't even really know, but who represented the possibility of your own metamorphosis. Twenty minutes into our first date, I had already begun picturing myself as his girl-friend, squired about town to farmers markets and cocktail bars and weekend brunches, not as a loner hiding behind a book but as someone's cherished partner. It wasn't the TV writer I was mourning—when I ran into him in a parking garage a few months later, I had to struggle to recall his name—but the loss of that version of myself, the one who was loved and desired (and thin, always thin) and who could casually slip "my boyfriend" into conversation, and the older I got, the further I felt I was getting from ever being able to.

In Nora Ephron's 1987 autobiographical novel *Heartburn*, newly jilted protagonist Rachel is helped onto a plane by a handsome foreign stranger and immediately begins to wonder whether he's single and/or turned off by Jewish women and/or willing to have his subcutaneous cysts removed for her, before sternly reminding herself of her "vow not to have marital fantasies about strangers." I saw myself in that line when I first read the book, but it wasn't the men I dated or crushed on that I readily fantasized about attaining; it was the evidence of their interest, the cold, hard proof that someone had deemed me worthy of loving. I'd lost the weight—as it turned out, that had been the relatively easy part—but the part of me that felt fundamentally unworthy was harder to shed (and anyway, like so many dieters, I didn't feel "done" once the scale reflected a certain number; all my forty- or fifty-pound weight loss had done was instill in me the self-competitive desire to lose even more).

If you'd asked me when I was twenty-three, I would have

told you that I was pushing ever forward with my dieting in an effort to meet the right guy. Now, though, I look back and wonder; was I actually diverting my attention toward dogged pursuit of Weight Watchers–approved glory so I wouldn't have to turn it toward a romantic partner? I'd never been in a real relationship, and the mechanics of it all were so shrouded in mystery. I knew how to go on a first date in a darkened bar, how to angle my newly bony knees to the side and prop my chin in my hand and ask questions about work and hobbies and siblings, but I had no idea how to actually *be* with someone, how to cross the dreaded intimacy bridge and find yourself intact at the other side. *How do you know how to act around them?*, I would wonder to myself when I saw random couples buying groceries or arguing about where to park, not so far removed from the sixth-grade girl who'd covetously eyed the boys filing into the school theater for co-ed play practice and wondered what on earth I was supposed to say to them. Was there some script I hadn't been issued?

I wanted a boyfriend then, of that I was sure. I wanted it more than anything, I told myself, but the bulk of my mental energy wasn't devoted to sending inventive OkCupid messages or joining singles' sports leagues; instead, it was spent on what I like to call "diet math," the confounding mental arithmetic that accompany Weight Watchers and so many similar diet plans. *Can I eat this muffin? Do I have enough points left? What will I have for dinner, and how bad will I feel about myself once I eat it? Do I have time to leave the office for an hour to hop on a treadmill and earn myself some more food? Does Ralphs still sell those seven-point granola bars, and if so, can I survive on one all day without passing out on the bike ride home?* It might all sound painfully prosaic, but trust me, it gets exhausting.

Meltzer, too, knows that particular brand of exhaustion, and it's one she's alternately willing to suffer through and unable to stomach for too long (especially in the midst of an unprecedented global pandemic, which has forced so many of us to reconsider what we are and are not willing to put up with from our jobs, our doctors, our friends, our acquaintances, and even ourselves). "I needed some time away from Weight Watchers, because I had been living and breathing it for a few years," says Meltzer of her most recent short-term breakup with the diet, and she, too, is familiar with the concept of using dieting as a shield to keep the more challenging parts of life—like dating—at bay. "Not to sound too woo-woo, but I think we all have our own hang-ups and issues, and for me, it's not shopping, it's not making friends, there are a lot of things I don't have trouble with, but dating is really hard for me, and has been my whole life."

I should have known before speaking to Meltzer that being overall satisfied with your life doesn't preclude the possibility of harboring insecurities—most people do, after all—but for some reason, that's been a hard lesson for me to learn, contemptuous as I've always been of life's gray areas. "I think you think that you're either the ugliest girl in the bar or the prettiest, but what if you were just . . . somewhere in the middle?" a friend mused to me once when I called them, late at night, to tearfully recount some boy-related slight I'd suffered at an overpriced beer garden in LA's Highland Park neighborhood. I have no memory of who the boy was, or why his rejection—real or perceived—triggered a crisis of self-confidence in me, but I still remember the odd freedom that my friend's words instilled in me. For years, I'd been convinced that there was something about my personality or, more likely, my appearance that was getting in the way of my romantic success, but maybe I wasn't "other," wrong, different, marked at birth for solitude and unhappiness; maybe I was just wrestling with a raging case of low self-esteem.

This is part of the fundamental irony of eating disorders, or maybe just of existing in a body; what everyone else sees on the outside bears little to no resemblance to what you feel yourself to be on the inside. When I finally landed a high-powered assistant job on a new Amazon dramedy at the end of my first year in LA, something should have clicked into place; I should have thanked any god available to me for giving me the opportunity that everyone in Hollywood—except the Scientology Center employees, and maybe even them—dreams of, or at least held my head a little higher when I walked down the street, but instead, I was a wreck, subsumed by my fears. I knew the ability to convincingly smile and nod my way through a twenty-minute interview didn't mean I was actually ready for the job I was about to embark on, which involved managing the schedules of two extremely busy showrunners without dropping any of the seemingly infinite balls they juggled on a day-to-day basis. I'd never been remotely organized, had always been the kid who turned in sloppy, dog-eared homework two days past the due date; I didn't wonder *if* I'd fail at this new opportunity, I wondered *how* I'd fail, and I ramped up my binge eating accordingly.

I learned a lot working on that show, from how to furnish a writer's room to how to roll network execs' calls while navigating through Glendale on a bike to what, exactly, a "gaffer" did, but the main skill I honed was secrecy when it came to bingeing. A

TV set is probably one of the best places on earth to pass off your raging eating disorder as "stress relief," for a variety of reasons, the most important one being that the executive powers that be compensate for long hours and substandard pay with a vast cornucopia of snack items. Food is everywhere, whether it's snacks on set or catered lunch for the writers, and when everyone around you is working until 4:00 a.m., alternating sips of sugary bottled Frappucinos with fistfuls of Doritos, talking about how they're "going to start eating better next season," it's easy to do it, too; to let your fixation with food become low-hanging fruit for bonding. The entire job of craft services is to make sure there's always a bounty of food on set, and their main focus was feeding stars, set builders, production assistants, teamsters, and other on-set crew who got more hard physical labor done in a day than I did in a month; there wasn't time to do enough inventory to notice if, say, a family-size serving of Cheddar Bunnies went missing between takes.

Despite the relative easiness of my role on the show, the job was significantly harder than any I'd held previously, way tougher than occasionally ordering coffee and organizing pens for the three laid-back guy writers on the web series I'd worked on last. My bosses, Dana and Darlene, were in charge of every last detail of the show, from handing in scripts to consoling overwhelmed actors to dealing with network and studio bosses who always seemed to call at 6:00 p.m. with "a few *tiny* changes," and I felt physically sick every time I forgot to confirm a doctor's appointment or dropped a call, convinced they'd regret hiring the ditzy millennial with zero office skills. If they'd been stereotypical TV showrunners, bro-y and obsessed with dick jokes and luxury cars, it might not have bothered me to be so totally useless at my job, but these were two funny and generous working moms who still made time to ask about my weekend after spending forty-eight straight hours in the edit bay; I didn't want to let them down, and I didn't want them to ever find out just how I *actually* spent my weekends (bingeing, with occasional breaks to be dragged to various beaches and dive bars by my small and extremely patient group of friends).

By the time the show was unceremoniously canceled in the fall of 2017, I'd learned a little bit about how to work a landline and manage a calendar, and a whole lot about how to compress my eating disorder into what scant time I had available to attend to it during a nonstop workday. I became a pro at sneaking into a bathroom stall and swallowing Twinkies and Uncrustables in a minimum of bites during hour-long "dinner breaks," texting with one hand while I unwrapped my sad bounty with the other. The craft services guys were incredibly kind dad types obsessed with feeding my bosses (and, by extension, me), and it brought me near tears to imagine them finding out how I devoured their gifts of expertly Saran-wrapped leftover turkey meatloaf, spanakopita, and dirty rice: alone in the front seat of the used Subaru I'd acquired halfway through the season, parked outside the production office on a shadowy stretch of pavement near the trash cans where nobody ever ventured, avoiding eye contact with myself in the rearview mirror as I gorged. I kept my weight down then by starving after bingeing, refusing to allow myself more than a sip of water as my body strained for some kind of equilibrium.

Working in television didn't give me an eating disorder,

any more than having divorced parents or moving around a lot as a kid did, but it did create a perfect environment for my bingeing—not to mention my tendency to avoid the parts of life that didn't come naturally to me—to flourish. While I worked on the Amazon show, I mostly eschewed dating, reasoning with myself that I'd never manage to sustain a relationship while working sixteen-hour days and ignoring the fact that approximately half of my potential dating pool was keeping the same hours on one TV show or another. I nurtured an obsession with a constitutionally unavailable drummer for over a calendar year, turning a few weeks of average sex (that I nonetheless thought was great, having little but blackout-drunk hookups to compare it to) and hastily prepared morning coffee into a romance of such epic and heartbreaking proportions that one after another of my friends eventually banned me from discussing it.

The great thing about a fake relationship is that it's consistent; it's always stable, never slipping out of your grasp, and in a strange way, you're always in control. Just as I dreamed of disappearing without a trace into the TV writer's setup adult life, or of having some unknown guy caress my hip bones and tell me I was getting too thin, I harbored elaborate fantasies of being a drummer's girlfriend, of following him on tour and hawking T-shirts at his concerts and leveling his groupies with the nonchalant power of my gaze and never being forced to question my role in the room, or in the world. (This particular drummer's band, which played energetic yet actively bad pop-punk to audiences of teens, wasn't particularly besieged by groupies, but I imagined them fearing me anyway.)

I've always been better at fantasy than reality, at least when it comes to love. Back then, I was great at mentally decorating a studio for two in the cool-yet-cheap part of town and hashing out the specifics of band-related interpersonal drama, but when it came to actually looking a guy in the eye and asking, "Do you remotely like me, or should I stop sleeping with you?"—I seized up. There was a brief, triumphant week at the beginning of my on-and-mostly-off year with the drummer when I didn't binge at all; in fact, I barely ate, my appetite diminished by dopamine in a way it never had been before. *This is what it's supposed to feel like,* I told myself as we sat in front of the TV at the house he was dog-sitting at for the week, our spoons dipping lackadaisically in and out of the tonkotsu broth I'd picked up for us at Silverlake Ramen as we watched *It Follows* and kissed between jump scares.

Now, with the benefit of hindsight, all I can think about is the fact that the drummer neither paid for nor picked up our ramen. (*He's tired from band practice, and plus, I have a steady paycheck,* I told myself, overlooking the fact that my salary was barely enough to afford the $600 monthly rent on the awkwardly tented one-bedroom I still shared with Jenna.) I was just so charmed, though, to have a guy to sit next to on the couch, a sad-cute, reasonably tall, floppy-haired guy of the kind I never thought I'd be playing footsie with during a horror movie I never would have watched on my own. I would have done anything to keep the drummer's interest, to keep myself the kind of girl who could take or leave a bowl of thick, salty ramen. When he finally decamped for San Francisco, sending me occasional texts that underutilized punctuation and eschewed specifics, I told myself I'd stay floaty, stay wanted, *stay skinny*, but soon his texts were coming fewer and farther between, and the cheap fried-rice joints and Postmated doughnut orders were right where I'd left them, waiting for me.

Things never officially ended with the drummer; there was a last time I saw him, of course, but I didn't expect it, and I stayed tethered to the version of myself I'd been with him for exponentially longer than anyone wanted me to. I'd gotten my first taste of romantic ease, of someone pulling me in closer, and when the rejection inevitably came, my hunger surfaced to meet me. Soon, I was bingeing weekly again, if not daily, as my job sputtered toward hiatus before ending abruptly. I started freelancing as a journalist, trying desperately to eke out an identity (or at least a living) with clicky listicles for women's websites while deriving most of my scant income from babysitting.

Taking care of kids is another red-hot opportunity for a binge eater. I'd had experience in the field back in Brooklyn, but LA babysitting was a whole different ball game. I lucked into the path of a gorgeous, blond, ex-Mormon woman with three kids who owned a palatial house in the Pacific Palisades with her equally gorgeous, blond, ex-Mormon husband; there were lemon trees in the front yard, a trampoline out back, and, in the all-white kitchen, a pantry stocked with every organic kids' snack sold at Whole Foods. Once I got the kids—eight, six, and one, all towheaded and charismatic and easy enough to wrangle—down for bedtime, I took up residence on the immaculate leather couch, chocolate milk in one hand and microwavable fish sticks in the other, watching whatever was on while I filled myself to bloating until I saw the headlights of the parents' convertible illuminating the dark of the driveway.

My time in Los Angeles gave me so much; a driver's license, a start to my not-so-illustrious dating career, a lifelong friendship with Eliza, and the building blocks of my work as a journalist number among my biggest acquisitions there. While it's the city that made me a reasonably independent adult, a writer, and a sexual being (very much in that order), it's also the place where I came to know the lowest depths of my life with food. In LA, I learned exactly how far I'd go—how many miles I'd drive, how many dollars I'd spend, how many plans I'd cancel, how many work commitments I'd bail on—to feed my addiction, and I formed a relationship with food that was compensatory, rather than celebratory. When I didn't get what I wanted, I ate, and soon enough, the food *became* the wanting; then, as now, they were inextricably bound up with one another.

I've never been thinner than I was when I shared that one-bedroom with Jenna off a busy West Jefferson Boulevard, and I may never be again, but even the knowledge that I'd been largely miserable during that part of my life didn't protect me from turning the era into a kind of mental Garden of Eden, a fixed time and place when I'd been skinny, and therefore wantable. I eventually came to understand that my fear of dating and my fear of fat were—are—linked, but still, part of me (the most therapy-resistant part imaginable) truly believed that if I wore a sample size, I was better off than I had been before I alternated binges with starvation that made me too dizzy and weak to speed-walk a block. Pretty stupid, right? Then why couldn't I turn it off for good?

Chapter 4

HOPE

In a Season 4 episode of the Netflix series *BoJack Horseman*, BoJack—the titular depressed cartoon horse guy—accidentally calls his half-sister Hollyhock a "blob" while he's trying to convince her to dump a superficial Hollywood poser. He's repeating the same word she used earlier that day, but it still smarts; later in the episode, Hollyhock asks BoJack "Do you ever get that feeling that to know you more is to love you less?" When I first watched that episode in late 2017, prostrate on my mattress in the tiny Highland Park bedroom I rented from an inordinately cheerful freelance photographer whose perpetual good mood seemed like nothing so much as a rebuke to my own sadness, I wanted to leap through the screen, grab Hollyhock by the shoulders, and scream "YES, I get that fucking feeling."

Everything else in LA seemed to be about physical beauty and artificial joy (or, at least, I had to believe everyone on social media's joy was artificial if I didn't want to feel even worse about myself), but here was someone who felt as wrong and ugly here—inside and out—as I did, even if she was a cartoon. I was between full-time jobs at the time, living off a shallow cache of assistant-job savings and babysitting money, and I would spend my days getting high alone in the back-yard and ordering Postmates hauls of doughnuts or Cheez-Its or pizza to my door, hoping the photographer and our other roommates would be out so they wouldn't see me doing the shuffle of shame back to my room with a decidedly nonsolo serving of food. Then I would lie prone on my mattress and eat, staring at Netflix with dull, empty eyes and avoiding calls from my parents, from Jazmine, from Eliza, and our other best friend from college, Natalie—pretty much from anyone who loved me. I couldn't face them, because then I would have to face myself.

"Pretend I have a broken leg," I remember imploring my friend Daniella, who had flown across the country from New York in the winter of 2018 for a visit and quite reasonably ex-pected to see me. I wanted so badly to get out of bed, wanted to hug Daniella and go to a concert with her at the Lodge Room and act like a normal person, but I just couldn't do it, couldn't do anything except watch TV and cram Reese's Peanut Butter Cups I could barely taste into my mouth by the handful. I felt like I had my sophomore year of college, when I'd hit my first diagnosed clinical-depression wall and spent an entire winter break staring out the window of my mom's empty apartment and wearing the same giant denim sack of a shirt every day until it was filthy, except the problem back then had had an eventual solution; 10 milligrams of Lexapro, which I'd steadily bumped up to 20 milligrams over the years. Now I was stymied; how could I be on meds and still be *this* miserable, worse than I'd ever felt before?

It's easy now to dismiss the pain I was in at twenty-three, to wallpaper over the fact that my misery back then was so acute it often seemed to take the shape of another person in my empty bedroom with me, peering over my shoulder and cruelly mocking me for being so weak. All my situational anxiety—over not being thin enough, not being a successful writer, not having enough friends in LA, feeling lonely all the time, never having been in love or come close or even had a guy properly ask me out—eventually settled into a bone-deep certainty that it wasn't my circumstances making me unhappy; it was me. I was convinced that everything bad that had ever happened to me—from my parents' divorce to my friends' eighth-grade abandonment to my many blurry, half-remembered sexual encounters in and after college—wasn't bad luck, it was *of* me, somehow, and the worst part was that I was acutely aware of just how many advantages I was squandering with my sadness. "All my parents want is for me to be happy, and I can't even give them that," I remember wailing to Eliza on one of the rare occasions I actually spoke to someone about what was going on inside me; even now, my heart aches to remember how guilty I felt for my own suffering.

I can't remember exactly what sequence of events led to me getting in my car and driving the thirty minutes or so to my first twelve-step food group meeting,* but I know it was around that time, maybe even later in that same winter of 2018, which means it would have been shortly after my disastrous second date with an all-around affable Twitter personality in his mid-thirties who traveled in exactly the kind of cool LA circles that had always eluded me. Our first date was at Good Luck Bar, a now-closed spot in Los Feliz that was, in retrospect, uncomfortably heavy on Asian-inspired decorative flourishes for a bar owned by two white dudes; I had learned to drive less than a year before, and I'd suggested the place primarily because it was across the street from a supermarket with a seldom-surveilled parking lot where I could leave my car without having to parallel park.

Twitter Guy and I had fun at Good Luck Bar, or at least I thought so, but when we went out a second time—this time to some random bar in Silver Lake for happy-hour drinks after work, which maybe should have been a sign that he Just Wasn't That Into Me—things were different. He seemed quiet and distant all night, which led to my acting quiet and distant all night, and then finally confronting him about whether or not he even liked me "like that," which led to me sobbing in the driver's seat of my Subaru while he tried in vain to gently let me down (a lot of emotional labor to expend on a girl you've never so much as kissed, I now realize). If you're reading this, Twitter Guy, sorry, and thanks for

---

* You may notice that throughout this chapter, I do not name my twelve-step recovery program. This is out of adherence to its principle of anonymity; even though I'm no longer actively in the program, I still want to respect its boundaries.

being kind to a deeply depressed twenty-four-year-old girl with no particular regard for herself.

At one point, Twitter Guy assured me that dating him would be awful, that he would put me through hell, to which I responded through tears, "I'm in hell all the time, anyway." I don't remember saying this. I only vaguely remember feeling it, but I know I did, because it's written out in a Notes app on my phone. At some point that night, Twitter Guy hugged me and got out of my car. At some other point that night, I, too, got out of my car and kept drinking elsewhere, which I don't remember doing, but I must have, because I blacked out, which isn't great, because I know I drove home; I know this because I remember coming to in my driveway surrounded by empty, grease-stained McDonald's bags, managing to be shocked at myself even from under a protective layer of booze and food-induced numbness.

When I think about the person I was at twenty-four, the person who chased unavailable older guys and drove through LA blackout drunk (even just once) and cried alone in her car and never, ever talked to anyone about her bingeing, I automatically think of my favorite paragraph from Meaghan O'Connell's essay "Now You Know," which I first encountered in the 2010 anthology *Coming & Crying*: "Ask me what I wanted to be then and I would have said a vessel, a landscape, to disappear. A smart girl a cool girl a girl who makes you forget your mother left you; a girl whose hand you never stop holding when you show her David Lynch movies for the very first time. I wanted to be down for whatever, to wear the right thing and let him take it off, so cool, while he bent me over the desk and fucked me without asking. I wanted to understand him, to save him, to not touch him afterward because I get that he just wants to stare up at the ceiling and laugh for a while after we high-five. I wanted him to take my hand to anywhere. I would have gone wherever."

I would have gone wherever, too, would have put myself through anything in order to jump past the confines of what I saw as my own sad, small life and into someone else's. I knew getting strung out over one guy or another was a rite of passage that more or less all my friends back in New York were going through, but even back then, the hurt and heartbreak I felt over my brief and ultimately failed romantic encounter with Twitter Guy felt unbearable, precisely *because* nothing had really happened; I felt like a fantasist, a scared and lonely kid doing an impression of a woman living an adult life. I burned with shame to imagine him telling his friends about me, the needy twenty-something he'd had to let down easy; I hated the idea of being pitied. Is that what pushed me to get in my car one weeknight in 2018 and drive to an unfamiliar high school campus in Pasadena and painstakingly locate Room 310 in the dark, all so I could sit in the company of other people with food issues—something I was just beginning to understand I had, too—and listen?

I don't think I talked at all at that first meeting, not even when the kindly facilitator asked in soft, encouraging tones if anyone was "new to the program." I sat in an uncomfortable plastic chair and fiddled with my jeans zipper and accepted a lot of literature, and that was pretty much it. For some reason, I went back; for some reason, I kept going back, not every day or even always every week, but often enough. For the first few months of the chunk of time I spent consistently going to meetings, it was the little things—the way the light hit the floor at one midday meeting; the skinny girl my age in the yellow raincoat who held a pen like a cigarette at another; the quiet, antiseptic kindness of two meeting attendees making small talk on the walk back to their cars—that moved me, not the big, God-shaped transformation I assumed people went to twelve-step meetings in order to undergo.

To be honest, the God vibe of the whole thing kind of unnerved me. I often thought of *SMILF*'s Bridgette quietly thanking "goddess" in her own food group, wishing I could screw up the courage to sub in "they" for "he" when I read aloud from the Big Book without feeling like an idiot. I liked the part of meetings where we went around and talked about what was going on with us in three-minute "shares," with someone—never me—volunteering to be timekeeper, but I dreaded the meetings that were devoted to Big Book study, which seemed to me to be not particularly relevant to disordered eating and to have been written with middle-aged, white, cishet male alcoholics in mind (which, when I first read Leslie Jamison's *The Recovering*, I learned was more or less true; what I also learned, though, and would soon experience firsthand in twelve-step meetings, was what Jamison called "the eerie intimacy of hearing myself spoken aloud").

At first, I didn't understand why the meetings had to be so regimented. They seemed to run on the skills of people (primarily women) who were infinitely better organized than I was, the kind of women who were once the girls who received straight

As and teacher-scrawled raves about perfect penmanship while I was blowing off homework and constantly losing my planner. Slowly, though, I began to see that for every group-leader type who organized the meetings and kept time and passed around the donation envelope to keep meetings running, there was someone who skirted through the door ten minutes after the meeting started, someone who shifted nervously in their seat or stole illicit looks at their watch or looked visibly uncomfortable with the bodily and mental presence that attending a meeting requires. In other words: I began to see there were people like me here, even if their circumstances looked completely different from mine, and I began to think that—as corny as it was—maybe we could help each other just by showing up.

As I attended more and more meetings all across LA, ruling some out for a mixture of stupid and genuine reasons—the parking at this one sucked, the proximity to a mall Cinnabon at another all but invited a binge, there was a guy at a third who drove me absolutely insane with irritation every time he spoke through absolutely no fault of his own—and eventually settling into a one- or two-meeting-per-week routine with a "home meeting" that focused on women, sexuality, and body image and met not too far from me every Thursday night, I started to understand, almost against my will, why the rules were so important. The thing about my recovery program—the thing about most twelve-step programs, I imagine—is that "program," as many attendees call it, doesn't care who you are; it just wants you to show up, sit down, listen, and try your best to be accountable. You share for three minutes, not four or five, because that's what the person before you did, and that's what the person after you will do, too; this kind of built-in equity spoke to me, and I began to hold new respect for the people who did the deeply unsexy work of giving new attendees literature and setting up outreach phone trees and all the other meat-and-potatoes homework associated with the extraordinary "roteness" of sobriety or abstinence.

"When you're here, you're family," I'd sometimes think on my way to or from a meeting, before remembering that that was actually the Olive Garden slogan. I'd spent my entire life studying and socializing within the kind of rarefied academic institutions that touted their "diversity" as an admissions-brochure selling point, but here was actual diversity, in race and ethnicity and size and gender and sexuality and socioeconomic background, all around me. All these people, most of whose lives were so very different from mine, shared one thing with me—when it came to food, they couldn't stop—and finding that kind of community, even under fluorescent lights in synagogue meeting rooms and ugly-wallpapered community centers, helped me as much in my recovery as anything has to date, even if it wasn't a permanent fix.

A lot of the time, the program was a chore—not only actually sitting through the hour, but locating a meeting on the glitchy website, figuring out how to get there, dealing with the stymieing mess of LA parking, getting through the door on time (something I was never particularly good at doing, no matter how often I reminded myself that being late displayed an unacceptable level of disrespect for my fellow meeting attendees' time and energy), sitting down, and actually, well . . . *being present*, rather than day-dreaming and wishing desperately that I could look at my phone. I went to meetings in much the same way that I ran around the Silver Lake Reservoir two or three times a week; awkwardly and resignedly, full of boredom but not without some measure of hope that if I just showed up for long enough, a sea change would take place within me.

I probably don't have to tell you that the sea change—like Godot—never came. There was never a day when I woke up feeling fully healed, but slowly, I began to look forward to meetings, not always (okay, not ever) as spiritual liberation, but sometimes just as a welcome event to break up the long days and nights I could never quite manage to fill. Eventually, I started working with a sponsor, a cool, cropped-haired woman in her mid-thirties who'd met her wife in a twelve-step program for alcohol recovery and had only come to identify food as her "cross addiction" once she'd gotten sober. She handed me my very own blue-bound copy of the Big Book to keep, one that still lives on my bookshelf despite my God-related reservations (which, it turned out, my sponsor shared), and encouraged me to write out a history of my life in food that ended up filling the better part of a notebook.

I wonder what my life, or at least that awkward, ungainly stretch of it, might have looked like if I'd stayed in the program, or at least kept in contact with my sponsor. I've thought a lot about what I gained from the six months or so that I "audited" meetings (the semi-derisive term for showing up to meetings without really "working the program," or making your way through the twelve steps) in LA, and the best description I can find comes from Mary Karr's *Lit*, a crackling 2009 memoir of the author and poet's journey toward sobriety as a young mother. At one of Karr's first twelve-step meetings, she—an agnostic, at the time—describes pugnaciously asking a fellow sober drunk, Janice, what she gets out of getting down on her knees to pray. Janice tells her, "It makes you the right size. You do it to teach yourself something. When my disease has a hold of me, it tells me my suffering is special or unique, but it's the same as everybody's. I kneel to put my body in that place, because otherwise, my mind can't grasp it."

The life I'd lived up to that point was not about making yourself "the right size" (in spiritual terms, anyway); my high school prized academic and social competition and single-mindedness, handing straight As and prized awards to the kids who worked relentlessly and never seemed to slow down, and even in college, the first place I remember feeling truly at home, I found my niche by reporting on goings-on around campus for the school blog, a job that required me to examine—and, inevitably, judge—the world around me with a keen eye for potential humor or newsworthiness. The program was the first place where I felt accepted, not because of some achievement of mine, not because I'd told the right joke at the right time or filed my web copy early or stayed up all night on Ritalin to struggle my way to a C+ on a math test, but *because* of the mess that I felt my life was at that point. I belonged there because of the terror and loss of control I associated with eating; my presence there was justified *stam*, a Hebrew word Jamison defines in *The Recovering* as "for no earthly reason: because because."

I showed up to meetings because it reminded me that I was,

existentially speaking, the same as the person in the seat next to me, no better and no worse. Outside the four walls of a meeting, I could carry on cruelly evaluating myself and everyone around me, but for that one or two or three hours a week, I was able to put my desperation aside and allow for at least the *possibility* of grace—for myself, and for everyone else in the room. Here, at long last, were the people who ate one handful of tortilla chips and found themselves creeping back into the kitchen at midnight for the rest, the people who heard "How about we stop for ice cream?" and felt fear and unbearable longing rather than joy, the people who cut their food into tiny pieces or pushed it around their plates or ate it all at once over the sink and ended up feeling bad about it regardless.

I think a lot these days about the ways in which people ask for help, and what kind of help is available to them when (or if) they do. For many, if not most, of us, it doesn't come naturally; we live under a capitalist system that valorizes self-reliance and independence, and we end up taking on that pressure as individuals, sure that our addictions and compulsions (or our poverty, or our disability, or our difficulty securing safe housing, or any other aspect of life that we're struggling with) is our own fault. I wish desperately we as a society learned to praise the act of reaching out for assistance as much as we do self-regulation and autonomy. Is there anything more vulnerable in this world than admitting you're not okay than outstretching a hand without knowing ahead of time whether anyone will be there to take it? Is there anything more brave than giving up on the fallacious notion that the only way to recover is to go it alone?

When I first watched the third-season episode of Rachel
Bloom and Aline Brosh McKenna's musical dramedy *Crazy Ex-
Girlfriend* in which protagonist Rebecca—played by Bloom—
attempts suicide via an overdose of pills on an airplane, I got
chills, not because of the attempt itself, but because of the scene
in which a bleary-eyed, increasingly out-of-it Rebecca briefly
sees the bright-red HELP sign above her airplane seat as reading
HOPE. In a small, weak voice, she calls over a flight attendant
who had been friendly to her earlier on, showing her the empty
pill bottle; Rebecca has more or less spent her entire existence
up to that point on her own, trying to prove her worth to her
hyper-critical mother by laser-focusing on work to the exclu-
sion of everything and everyone around her, but she saves her
own life in that moment by admitting that she *can't* do it alone.
Sometimes help looks like hope, and vice versa; sometimes you
can't summon the latter without admitting how desperately you
need the former.

I've turned to a lot of sources for help defining my relationship with food and eating in the years since I fell out
of the habit of going to meetings regularly, but the lodestar
I've looked to most often is Laurie Colwin, the *Gourmet* food
columnist and fiction writer who died in 1992 at the age of
forty-eight. I've devoured Colwin's food writing so ravenously
over the years that I can all but hear her voice in my head as I
read, telling me to splurge on the good olive oil at the grocery
store (or, conversely, not to bother buying a fancy loaf pan,
because you can reliably pick them up for cheap at almost
any garage sale). Most of Colwin's cooking advice is cheerily

practical and frill-free, but one of my favorite quotes of hers from the 2000 book *More Home Cooking* reads like a motto for how to conduct yourself in *and* out of the kitchen: "We know that without food we would die. Without fellowship, life is not worth living." Colwin makes a passionate case for sharing food, home-cooked or store-bought, with the people in your life, and her reference to "fellowship" reminds me that eating in the company of loved ones isn't just an exercise in caloric absorption, it's a daily undertaking with the potential to tether us ever more tightly to the people around us, not unlike, say, the practice of attending a twelve-step meeting.

It was always the fellowship of my food group that I craved, after all, not the spiritual component (or, rather, fellowship *was* the spiritual component for me; to this day, I'm far more comfortable locating the divine in the collective than anywhere else). In Colwin's writing, I began to see that I could keep finding commonalities with others around food—in its preparation, its consumption, even its outsize importance in my life and the terror that my craving for it often instilled in me— without the organizing system of a meeting bolstering me. She didn't make having a good relationship with food and eating seem simple, exactly; she admitted that cooking takes work (and that finding fresh, nutritious ingredients to prepare food with has always been easier for some people than others) but she also stressed that it was work worth doing, for yourself if for no one else.

Talking to Leslie Jamison—the aforementioned author of *The Recovering* as well as four other books—about addiction, compulsion, and recovery on a recent weekday felt a little like a JV player chatting up Michael Jordan, but as we spoke on the phone while Jamison made the trek to pick up her child from school, I was reminded of the unspoken undercurrent of sameness that so often travels between two people who have familiarity with the format of a twelve-step meeting (and, more broadly, those who know what it's like to live with an eating disorder). I'd read Jamison's account of her encounter with anorexia as a young adult in *The Recovering* and been awed by how word-perfectly she described the sensation of living a shrunken life, the parameters of which were drawn by food, but once we began to talk about what we liked—and didn't—about group-based eating-disorder recovery, it felt very much like I was meeting up for coffee with anyone from the Thursday-night home meeting where I'd first gotten comfortable with the program back in LA in 2018.

"There were a thousand differences between eating-disorder recovery and booze recovery for me," Jamison recalls of her own journey toward sobriety and abstinence, explaining: "With food, my issue was restriction, not abundance, and I couldn't just eliminate the concrete thing from my life and *then* start to deal with all the complicated psychological stuff around its removal—which was what I did with booze. I knew food was going to have to be a part of my life every single day for the rest of my life. The difference between those two processes taught me that recovery can look many different ways, even if it always has to involve some daily, constant, ongoing reckoning."

This kind of reckoning, which is referred to in some recovery circles as "a searching and fearless moral inventory" ("*Oh, okay, NBD, I'll get right on that*," I jeered sarcastically in my head when I first heard the term, unused as I was to making moral inventories of any kind, searching and fearless or otherwise), often feels like the absolute last thing I want to do when I'm hungry and tired and more in the mood to stuff infinite Goldfish crackers into my mouth than analyze the deeper meaning behind my sudden desire for a snack. I remember bringing this up at one of my twelve-step meetings in LA at the very beginning of my recovery process, desperately asking the room if I could ever expect to eat normally again.

Nobody chimed in—they weren't supposed to, per the "no-crosstalk" rule—but if they had, I would imagine they might have asked me what "eating normally" looked like to me. It would have been a good question, and I wouldn't have had an answer; all I knew then was that I wanted to free myself of the newly ac-quired burden of knowledge of my own compulsion, desperate as I was to find a way out of what I saw as the life of cautious, carefully measured, inventory-based food intake stretching out endlessly before me. I wanted freedom, spontaneity, the license to dispense with the rules I was just starting to learn; as grateful as I was for the fellowship of my weekly meeting, I didn't think that was something it could ever grant me.

There was an explicit "no diet talk" rule at my weekly meet-ing, but diet brain always seemed to find a way to creep in re-gardless. The other women in my Thursday-night group had cut out sugar, fat, caffeine, carbs, sodium—anything and everything to avoid coming into contact with their "trigger foods"—and I didn't doubt that each of them was the best judge of what worked for their own recovery, but all that avoidance reminded me uncomfortably of Weight Watchers. I knew we were all here to untangle our knotted relationships with food, but underneath that clearly stated goal, I was dimly aware of the same pulsing, unspoken desire for thinness that had propelled the sixth-grade girls at my middle school to subsist on nothing but one ice cream sandwich a day. Maybe it was unrealistic to expect that that slenderness obsession wouldn't follow us, but I couldn't help feeling disappointed when it did.

I kept coming back, though, week after week, just like they tell you to, and eventually I began to crave the ritual—not as much as I craved large amounts of food eaten alone between the four walls of my bedroom, or nights in my car in quiet parking lots, but enough to actually get me to meetings. "Part of what was important to me about fellowship and recovery was that it helped me feel like my life wasn't just losing something. It had something in it that it hadn't had before; very concretely, it had these meetings, these spaces, these folding chairs, these voices, these human stories," recalls Jamison, and I remember anchoring myself to those same details, desperate for a sense of community (even if it was community formed around the eating habits I was so miserably ashamed of) to supplant the bone deep loneliness that had come to encircle me during my time in LA.

For a relatively long time, fellowship truly did work for me, pulling me out of the miserable mire of my own self-loathing and solipsism long enough to remind me that there were people all around me who understood what I was wrestling with and wanted to help me. Slowly, I began to let my friends and family back in, if not fully—back then, I would sooner have left the house fully naked than admitted to anyone the quantity and quality of food I was gorging myself on, not to mention the cost of said food that had my bank account reserves dwindling by the day—then at least partly. I started returning Natalie and Eliza and Jazmine and my parents' calls, sometimes to vent and sometimes just to listen, newly aware that I hadn't been doing much of the latter over the past year or so. (At the time, I hadn't been aware that Eliza was in regular touch with Jazmine to talk about how to handle my obvious depression, with the two of them even reaching out to my dad for advice when things got particularly bad.)

I stopped dating (not that I'd really been doing much of it in the first place since the Twitter Guy debacle) and started ordering inexpensive moisturizers and serums on K-beauty sites, gently patting them into my skin and staring at myself in the mirror of the shared bathroom in the Highland Park house, hoping to like what I saw. "It's all about stopping and pausing and asking for your Higher Power's will," a fellow attendee reflected at one meeting, and I dutifully copied the phrase into my journal in the parking lot after I left. I dug my nails into the steering wheel of my car as I drove home that day, my whole body gripped by a desperate desire for strength; the strength to stop, to pause, to consider how a binge would make my mind and body feel before diving in instead of numbing out and waking up in the morning full of nausea and shame. A lot of the time, I still couldn't summon the particular strength not to pull up Postmates and place a binge-food order; when I could, it felt electrifying, like there was nothing in the world I couldn't conquer.

I'd always been the kind of person who scoffed at affirmations (read: sort of an asshole), but when one of my favorite fellow attendees at my Thursday-night meeting slipped me a list of statements to recite to myself "as often as you need to," I found myself smiling and thanking her in a low tone of voice that didn't feel totally disingenuous. The statements ranged from the expected ("I am beautiful") to the ED-specific ("I deserve to eat until I feel full and nourished and stop when I'm ready"), and I dutifully copied each affirmation into my journal, often with the mid-'90s yowl of Alanis Morissette—herself an eating-disorder survivor—playing through my earbuds as I did so. I listened to Morissette's 1995 song "Not the Doctor" on my cracked iPhone constantly throughout that strange season of my life, exulting in the lyric that made me feel most seen: "I don't want to be your food or the light from the fridge on your face at midnight, hey / What are you hungry for?"

"If mental health were as easy as repeating mantras, wouldn't everyone just do that?" I groused to Eliza one night, but I was living in LA, the home of manifestation and positive energy and claiming your miracles; didn't I owe it to myself to try? I felt like a colossal idiot at first, repeating my affirmations out loud to myself in the mirror in a flat, neutral voice during skincare time, but I did it anyway; not every day, not even every other day, and not always in the moments when I most needed the confidence, but often enough that it felt like the beginning of something.

"Better" meant something different to me when I first started the program; I knew I couldn't keep living with my binge eating like this, either the act of it or its inevitable, wrecking aftermath, but could sooner imagine myself sprouting wings than attaining genuine bodily peace—much less living my life as a resignedly fat person. (I now think: *How could I have, really, when that image had never been modeled for me? It was easier to wish myself thin than to imagine myself fat and truly happy.*)

When I read Jessica Knoll's description of traumatized, razor-sharp striver Ani FaNelli limiting her binge eating to "Sundays, and the occasional Wednesday night" in the 2015 novel *Luckiest Girl Alive*, I felt a shiver of recognition: I was so sure then that I could only be safe if I disappeared into a life of women's-magazine bylines and gleaming engagement rings like Ani did at the book's outset, evidence stacked up all around me that I was smart, attractive, wantable, my desperate and out-size craving for binge food contained safely within a set of rules that let me have my peanut butter (I, like Ani, had binged on jars of it regularly since childhood, craving its rich, starchy nothingness) and eat it, too.

In retrospect, I know there were people in my recovery program who were closer to Laurie Colwin than Ani FaNelli in their individual approaches to food. There were definitely fat people at my meetings, fat people who talked about partners and kids and jobs and travel and friendship as casually and unremarkably as anyone else, but I was still thin then; my eyes didn't immediately triangulate the location of any other fat person in the room as a potential source of support, and I still thought on some level that to be fat was somehow to live your life at a quieter, lesser decibel than a thin person would (no matter how boldly I had proclaimed otherwise all over the various comments sections of the feminist blogosphere for years).

Was there fatphobia present in my meetings? Of course—after almost thirty years of life, I have yet to enter a space totally free from its long shadow—and although it felt like something each of us brought along with us, rather than something created by the space itself, I eventually started to feel caged in meetings, like I just couldn't sit through one more person's account of their successful rejection of the doughnut box passed around at work without screaming. Although Jamison has gained much from fellowship around sobriety from alcohol, she's not insensible to its potential pitfalls within the context of disordered eating. "I'm twenty years out from the worst part of my disordered eating, and I still feel uncomfortable and triggered if someone is sharing about eating in a really restrictive way," Jamison explains, adding: "I feel critical and antagonistic, but I don't like feeling that way; I feel like an eighteen-year-old again. Because I'm constantly forging a relationship with food on a daily basis, I think I feel more vulnerable to the ways in which that relationship could be destabilized."

"Vulnerable" was the perfect description of how I felt in meetings, but I *wanted* to be destabilized. I wanted to gnash my teeth, to flail, to scream about my terror around food, to show everyone the ugly underbelly of what I was grappling with; the late-night food orders that the delivery person must have assumed were for a family, the pathetic retches in the sink the next morning, the red eyes and not-so-slowly shrinking savings account and the shame that I was sure emanated from me cartoonishly like a stench after I binged. Somehow, though, every time it became my turn to share, I found myself sanitizing my binges, sketching out vague details of my attempts to cook healthy and go for daily walks and always ultimately promising my fellow attendees I was "on the mend." (Why? Why did I feel the need to lie to strangers as much as I lied to the people in my life who loved me?) It felt like there were two Emmas, the one who binged and the one who went to meetings in an attempt to course correct, but I couldn't figure out how to fuse them.

I got a job around that time, another temporary assistant gig on a web series that conflicted with my regular Thursday-night meeting, and I know that was the more immediate reason for my cessation, but underneath that practical excuse was a layer of dissatisfaction I'd always felt but couldn't quite name: not with meetings, necessarily, but with the version of myself who existed in meetings, who drove there weekly with every intention of un- burdening myself but found it harder and harder to do so. Hearing other people's truths helped—of course it did, if only in making me feel less alone—but I began to feel uncomfortably like an energy vampire, sucking up other people's narratives of pain and addiction and loss of control when something always stopped me from accessing the emotional honesty necessary to be transparent about my own. I was no longer content with showing up, with being counted, with slowly cutting out sugar or carbs or whatever trigger food and learning to live a life within the confines of my own fear of excess; I wanted more from my recovery, but I didn't know back then what "more" might look like.

What happened next was both simple and not. I crashed my car, a 2010 Subaru handed down to me by my dad, and left LA for

New York a month or two later, using the money paid out to me by my insurance company (which should have rightfully gone to my dad, who was somehow generous enough never to stake his claim) to pad my landing. I've told the story for years now, playing it up for laughs—"I was speeding to a 4:20 showing of *Tully*, and then I went downhill and hit someone's parked car, and then this angel in jean shorts came outside and told me that it was *his* car, but not to worry"—and indeed, it began to seem funny later, the 4:20 showing and the speeding to a forgettable movie and the kind, shirtless stranger whose car had sustained a significant dent, but had indeed been fine. He'd been so sweet to me, reminding me to breathe as I sobbed and apologized and Googled the number of a tow company with shaking fingers; all these years later, I'm still amazed at his warmth to a stranger who'd carelessly damaged his property. I didn't feel I deserved it, but I needed it all the same.

At the time, though, with my car totaled and a bloody, oozing gash on my chin where I'd hit the steering wheel, I didn't realize how lucky I was (to be alive, to be mostly unhurt, to have parents who looked out for me while still allowing me to perform independence, to *walk away with money*. Who did that ever happen to after a car crash?). I'd been thinking about leaving LA for a while, even moving out of the Highland Park house and subletting my friend Olivia's room in a drafty, light-filled bungalow in Silver Lake while I "figured out my next move," but it took a text from Jazmine to give me the final permission I needed to change my life in a way that felt—however much my loved ones assured me it wasn't—like failure.

I'd long needed my friends to act as mirrors, reflecting my

own depression back to me in a way I actually had to acknowledge. Sophomore year of college, Eliza strode into my dorm room during the long period where I got out of bed only to microwave cups of neon-yellow Easy Mac and told me bluntly: "You seem miserable, dude." I *knew* I was miserable, knew it wasn't normal to skip so many classes and stay in bed all day and find joy in approximately nothing, but hearing it out loud turned it into something real, something I couldn't ignore. I'd been running on empty in LA for months, if not years, bingeing and hiding and crying and self-destructing in slow motion, and finally, when Jazmine texted me to suggest I move home to New York ("you can always go back to la after a while!"), I was ready to listen.

I didn't bring much to New York with me, just a duffel bag of clothes and another one filled with the twenty or so books from my collection that I hadn't left at my friend Hannah's house for safekeeping on the spurious notion that I'd eventually be back for them once I'd "gotten my head on straight." (Where did I come up with that 1950s-era, tough-it-out term?) I don't remember my flight out of LAX, or the moment I showed up on my mom's doorstep, or how it felt to have LA in my rearview mirror, but I know I brought my affirmations with me, printed out on the very same water-stained sheet of paper I'd been handed in that meeting months before. I wasn't reading them aloud to myself much anymore, but I kept that paper folded and tucked inside the red notebook I carried everywhere, just in case. You never know when you'll need to remind yourself of who you are—or, in my case, who you're trying to be.

Chapter 5

GORGE

If there's one thing every single fiction author and screenwriter loves, it's the "sad girl lands in New York and attempts to become a new person" trope, but when I arrived on the threshold of my new apartment in Brooklyn after a sweaty, aimless month in my childhood bedroom uptown, I wasn't hoping to wholly reinvent myself; I didn't expect to get that lucky. I just wanted to pay less than $1,000 for a room (I made it, just barely) and let the company of my college friends remind me who I'd been before I sank beneath the undertow of my depression and binge eating, before trying to meet new people or find stable work I liked, before even just filling my days in LA had begun to feel like hurling my body against a locked door.

My mom's first order of business upon my arrival was to nag me into making an appointment with a nonterrible psychiatrist who immediately prescribed Abilify, a brand-new drug that I was initially afraid to say yes to due to its classification as an "atypical antipsychotic." My doctor assured me that the label didn't mean *I* was psychotic, but she did inform me that I exhibited some signs of bipolar II disorder that had likely been hiding undiagnosed beneath a top layer of clinical depression for years. A low dose of Abilify would supplement my Lexapro, she promised, kick-starting the antidepressant that had once gotten me out of my dorm room bed and into the world and granting me the energy to vaguely enjoy my life again; if I gave my body time to adjust, she was sure I'd start seeing results. (Did I tell her about my bingeing? I must have, but I don't have any memory of her telling me about potential weight gain from Abilify; later, I'd rack my brain for it, sure she must have warned me.)

While I waited for the meds to make me happy, or at least happy-*ish,* I found a place to live, a surprisingly roomy apartment in Prospect Heights where the heat seldom worked right and mice were a monthly—if not weekly—reality, and where I would live in the smallest (and thus most affordable) bedroom, but with plenty of natural light and three older, cooler, surprisingly friendly people who'd all been seniors at my college when I was a first-year. I started refining my résumé, hoping that the scant months I'd put in working at a Los Angeles–based news and entertainment website before its billionaire CEO summarily shut the site down would convince *someone* to call me in for an interview. (In case it didn't, I was also ready to trump up the work I'd done on contract for the women's-interest digital media site where I'd filed a handful of stories to a kindly editor before *he* got laid off, making it sound like my Kardashian blogs and aggregated skin-care tips actually amounted to something worth mentioning.)

Right around the time the Abilify was settling in my system

for good, I landed a job—not a permanent one, and not one in journalism, but a temp gig on the nebulously named "Arts and Culture" team of a mononymous search-engine giant that a friend's friend was vacating for a better opportunity. Every morning, I took the C train from the Clinton-Washington stop by my apartment to Fourteenth Street and spent the following eight hours at a clean white desk, trying to figure out how to look busy. My boss was used to dealing with tech people who'd crunched raw data in college rather than writing bad autofiction, and whose work projects were accordingly complex; I think she was just too busy to realize that she was giving me as much time to, say, write a location blurb—"Low-key, cash-only tavern with a '70s vibe"—as she gave my numbers-facing colleagues to . . . well, do whatever it is they did with numbers.

I began to spend my vast, blank expanse of work hours trawling Twitter for pitch calls and doing my best to draft winning hed/dek/text combos, slowly placing stories across a variety of publications and—more importantly, and even more slowly—learning not to take it personally when the vast majority of those pitches were ignored. Nights I spent with my college friends, delighting in how easy it was to *do things* in New York; if I wanted to smoke weed and watch reality TV with Natalie, or read our respective books at a wine bar with Jazmine, or go see a screening of *Dog Day Afternoon* at BAM with my college friend Gavin, all I had to do was text them, and if someone couldn't meet up, I didn't take it as a personal slight the way I would have if a new friend bailed on me in LA.

I even started to meet new people, taking the bus to Williamsburg weekly for spin classes with my friend Kate from the college blog and her new friend Maya, all of us loudly dreading the forty-five-minute workout but admitting to one another at the juice place or the slice shop afterward that we felt disturbingly good. Kate and Maya both worked in media full-time, but they were—and this is crucial—not dicks about it, complaining about work at dive-bar happy hours around Brooklyn in ways that felt genuine rather than show-offy and offering to introduce me to editors and other writers who might be able to help me string more clips together. Suddenly, we were something of a trio, and I remembered that I actually *did* know how to make friends when I wasn't in a depressive spiral. I could feel the loneliness of the past year abating, loosening, the way shoulders do after a good stretch; I was still self-critical and prone to tears, not to mention regularly jumpy and nauseous from the Abilify, but I was starting to feel vaguely like myself again.

Dating women happened suddenly, or, looked at another way, after twenty-five years of denial. I'd first voiced my suspicions about my sexuality to Natalie in the stairwell of our freshman dorm, but I don't consider that a coming-out; I was half a year into my tentative campus reinvention, still acclimating to the idea of myself as a person with friends (plural), and when I told Natalie I thought about girls sometimes, I was more looking for confirmation that I was normal—read: straight— than anything else. There was no room within my conception of myself at that time for the confusing, stomach-twisting feelings I'd first felt for Meg from *Hercules* as a kid. I pushed them down instead, buried them with pizza and beer at frat parties to sublimate a desire I wasn't sure how to name. The queer community at my college intimidated me, and by the time I graduated, I still identified as "unsuccessful heterosexual" more than anything else. "If I were gay, I'd know it," I'd say frequently, submitting as evidence the fact that half my friends were queer; some of the time, I believed it.

In the years following college, I'd occasionally voice aloud to friends that I might *eventually* date women, but I didn't communicate any urgency to act on it. I don't remember changing my "Preferences" setting on Tinder, but I must have, because shortly before I left LA, I'd ended up on a first date with a woman named Lucy at a wine bar by my sublet. Lucy was sweet and cool, short-haired and artsy and into tarot before it was everywhere, and when we made out in her car, it wasn't an instant confirmation that I'd been gay all along (back then, I was still naive enough to think those kinds of epiphanies existed for all "real" gay people), but I remember thinking somewhere in the deep recesses of my consciousness: *Hmm.* I don't think I told my friends about the date with any particular significance—I know I called my dad and casually told him I'd gone on a date with a girl the night before, because I remember his surprisingly validating lack of follow-up questions—but all these years later, I'm still proud of myself for taking the risk, for changing my settings, for kissing a girl in a car and letting myself enjoy it (particularly at a point in my life where I'd all but forgotten how to enjoy anything).

I felt stupid coming out at twenty-four when most of the friends I thought of as *actually* queer had been out since high school, so stupid that I didn't officially do it; I even dated a cis-het guy during my first few months in Brooklyn, and I vaguely remember crying when we broke up, but I also remember that occasion dovetailing with the beginning of my girl-crazy era, which Amanda Richards—another queer digital-media writer who came out later in life, and someone who I now think of as a friend but first met on a dating app, if you need a hands-on demonstration of how small even the relatively expansive New York City queer community can be—memorably described thus in an *InStyle* article: "The red-hot glow of messy lesbian dating calls to me, and it feels impossible not to reach out and touch."

I played "Flirting with Her" by Sir Babygirl on repeat that fall and winter as I ran in Prospect Park and browsed the queer fiction section of my favorite used bookstore on Vanderbilt and binged as seldom as I had in college (for a few months, anyway), exulting in the song's frenetic beat and its overtly gay lyrics: "She left her name on my lips / I don't think I'll ever get over her hips / Or ever feel like anything else exists / When she texts me 'hey.'" (When I play that song now, I don't associate it with any of the myriad women from that time who captured my attention and ultimately curved me; instead, it brings me right back to finding myself at the center of a swirling mass of queer bodies on the dance floor, and being too brand new and unjaded—and, okay, drunk—to take any of it for granted. I'd pile myself into a Lyft Line in the wee hours, sweaty and glitter-streaked and mentally crafting a DM to whatever cute girl I'd met at the function, and come home and sleep until afternoon the next day, when I'd Seamless myself a cream-cheese-smothered hangover bagel and begin putting together that night's plans.)

Largely thanks to Twitter, I'd found a toehold in New York

media by the time I started dating women in earnest. Rachel Tashjian, a young editor from *GARAGE Magazine*—*Vice*'s (now-shuttered) art and fashion vertical—who had been a Twitter mutual for a while DM'd me about the possibility of interviewing for a soon-to-be-vacant assistant editor role when I was only halfway into my six-month contract at the search giant. I lied to my boss about a doctor's appointment, fished the only halfway-presentable shoes I owned—a pair of high-heeled black clogs that hurt my feet—out of the back of my closet, and took the train to DUMBO to interview at the office one afternoon, gleefully availing myself of *Vice*'s readily available kitchen stash of pretzels and hummus on the way out. (I still hold that the day I pass on free media-company-provided food is the day a light will truly go out inside me, even though its omnipresence at work is a daily binge trigger for me; who can ever really resist abundance?)

Everyone Rachel introduced me to at *GARAGE* looked more aptly dressed for a night of clubbing in Berlin than a day at the office, a fact that I tried not to let intimidate me too much as I agonized over my edit test; I felt strangely proud of the end result, though, and it must have gone over well, because I was offered the job a few days after I filed it. I promptly quit my temp gig and started as an assistant web editor at *GARAGE* in September 2018. Overnight, I went from drafting unpublishable personal essays on another company's time to writing as many as three or four articles a day for a site that was well known in the media world for mostly letting you write what you wanted, no matter how weird it was (unless, of course, it dinged an advertiser).

It was a lot of output, and I ended up burning out relatively quickly, but each day presented a new opportunity to write something potentially good and actually have people—a few people, at least—read it. The print side of the magazine confounded me, but I faked familiarity with terms like "TOC" and "the well" until I had the opportunity to steal away and covertly Google them. I did the same kind of panicked research with back issues of *Vogue*, quizzing myself on Marine Serre's signature print (crescent moons) and the pronunciation of Prabal Gurung (pruh-bal, like "trouble") until I could get through a pitch meeting without humiliating myself.

That fall also coincided with the start of my relationship with Jen, a wry, waifish mid-thirties magazine editor whom I'd met on Hinge. Our first date was at a conspicuously grown-up bar in Brooklyn with a fireplace and real tableware, an objective upgrade from the Jell-O-shot-slinging dive down the street where I still regularly caroused with my twenty-five-year-old friends until the wee hours, but I don't remember feeling intimidated by Jen's age and sophistication (or, rather, having never slept with a woman before, Jen's age and sophistication were low on the list of things I was worried about; mostly, I didn't want to be caught out as a fraud, a fake gay who'd kissed one girl in one car one time and decided to waste a *real* lesbian's time for mere exploration). When Jen and I made out outside the grown-up bar, though, it didn't feel like exploration; when she took me back to her sweet, tidy apartment, I suddenly forgot to feel stupid, turning my focus instead—maybe for the first time—to the person beside me in bed.

Did I feel insecure about how much smaller Jen was than me

that fall, as my hangover bagels added up and late-night binges started becoming a regularity for me again and I slowly began to gain weight—first in my thighs and stomach, then everywhere else? I'm sure I did, on some level; before coming out, I'd even trotted out my body issues as a reason why I couldn't *possibly* be a lesbian, telling Jazmine, "I feel like I'd just be comparing bodies with any girl I hooked up with." Jen and I dated for a few months, and when we broke up amicably and I began the painstaking, dating-app-fueled process of making up for lost time in terms of queer sex, I was too fueled by lust and confusion and hormones to mentally recite the daily litany of all the things that were wrong with my physical form.

During that first flush of girl-craziness, I don't remember ever holding a woman around the waist and wishing mine were leaner, or seeing someone else's jeans strewn on my bedroom floor and noting the smaller-than-mine size with chagrin. (This had happened to me before, with the sad drummer I'd wasted so much time on in LA; I remember mistakenly pulling on his black Levi 501s instead of mine one bleary-eyed morning and realizing with rising panic that they wouldn't stretch above my thighs. I would never have said anything to him, but I know I didn't put milk in my coffee that morning, too fearful of the calories.)

Ultimately, my relationships with Jen and the queer people who came after her were an exercise in slowly learning to be seen—to tolerate it and, eventually, even to like it—after a lifetime of longing for bodily disappearance; ironic, really, since the no-cishet-men-allowed dating app I used most often didn't even allow you to post photos of yourself. Users had the option of linking to their Instagram, but the first thing anyone saw about you was the brief message you'd compose, and for the first time, the insecure writer nerd within me thrived in a dating context. I might not have been physically arresting enough to get a ton of play on Tinder, I told myself, but I could certainly put together a two-hundred-word description of myself that would entice extremely online queers to message me. (I ended up doing a lot of the messaging, but I realize in retrospect that was something I needed; I'd spent my entire dating career frozen like a statue, waiting for the right guy to bring me to life, and I needed to climb down off my own pedestal and start to build up the layer of protective skin that comes with rejection. Pursuing women felt different, somehow, from chasing guys; it flipped the script I'd been given long ago about what it meant to be desirable, creating space for me to separate out what I actually wanted from what I'd been taught to want.)

Unconsciously, I'd long thought of the lesbian dating scene as somehow "easier" than the straight one from an aesthetic perspective, never forgetting ultra-nasty PTA mom Celia Hodes's rejoinder to her plus-size daughter Isabelle after catching her kissing a girl on the show *Weeds*: "You *cannot* become a lesbian just because you don't want to lose weight. The only girl that you should be seeing is Jenny Craig." I'd watched all of *The L Word* back in LA at the urging of my queer couple friends Lillian and Olivia, noting how impossibly, heartbreakingly thin the show's main heartthrob Shane McCutcheon was. By the time Jen and I broke up and I was officially on the lesbian market, I'd been steeped enough in queer pop cultural lore to know I wasn't a Shane—I was maybe more akin to an Alice or even an athletically challenged Dana—but one look at Shane's xylophone of a rib cage as she ripped the clothes off her hookup du jour still made me nauseous with insecurity, a feeling akin to unearthing my mom's press passes in high school. *Oh, right,* this *is what I'm supposed to be.*

I knew that the 2019-era Brooklyn counterpart to the aughts WeHo scene that Shane and her friends inhabited couldn't possibly be some Dionysian bacchanal of self-love and bodily acceptance, where weight was never an issue, but I was still crushed when I started attending Instagram-advertised queer parties and pop-up nights and noticed that the sexual dynamics therein often mirrored what I'd hated about straight nightlife, with the thinnest, whitest, most conventionally attractive queers receiving the lion's share of the attention. (Now, of course, I realize I was just going to the wrong parties, but I didn't know then how much more there was to being an out dyke in New York than trying and failing to successfully flirt with the hot mulleted bartender at The Woods on Wednesday nights.)

I started coaxing my small but mighty crew of lesbian friends into going to The Woods and Mood Ring and Nowadays and other queer or queer-adjacent clubs regularly, where I'd spend whole nights trying to catch a random girl's eye on the dance floor and feeling like shit when she never looked my way, my new exoskeleton of sexual confidence barely obscuring the bone-deep insecurity that was starting to rise to the surface. Daniella and our friend Brett, who'd both been out since college, would assure me that this was normal, that everyone struck out (and, more to the point, that not every queer person had to be a success on the club scene), but I hated losing the golden glow of newness that I had felt surrounding me when I first came out, insulating me from what I interpreted as my body *still* not being good enough to net me the things I wanted.

I was convinced I wasn't supposed to feel bad about myself anymore—wasn't that the whole point of coming out?—but I still did, and on some level, I think I resented my newfound queerness for not being able to shield me from a life's worth of accrued body issues. If being queer was the "answer" I'd searched for my whole life, the reason I'd never felt comfortable dating (or longing to date) guys, the hidden explanation for why I'd thought so incessantly about Meg and ADA Casey Novak from *Law & Order: SVU* and that one sixth-grade teacher of mine, then what did it say about me that coming out couldn't fix the problem that affected me most?

I now know that what I was experiencing was what activist and poet Sonya Renee Taylor refers to in her 2018 book *The Body Is Not an Apology* as "meta-shame," or "the state of feeling shame for feeling shame about our bodies." Taylor freely admits that this state of being is exhausting, and that's exactly how I'd describe it: the queer people I admired most on Instagram and at dance parties and Sapphically inclined happy hours didn't seem remotely concerned with thinness (at least to my untrained eye), but I still craved it, and I resented myself for craving it. I was reading a lot that year, burying my nose in this or that novel for the entirety of my morning commute to Dumbo via the B69 bus or bringing a galley of next season's buzziest book from work straight to MeMe's Diner, the queer restaurant two blocks from my apartment with the disco ball hanging kitschily from the ceiling. I'd settle at the counter and devour books and food in equal measure, allowing myself the all-American cheese puffs and patty melts and Hostess Sno-Ball-inspired cakes of the day that I would once have eaten only in a binge context and exulting in my communal, blissful, distinctly queer-feeling solitude. (It feels corny to say that MeMe's sparked the beginning of my spotty and deeply nonlinear healing process around food and queerness, but it also feels distinctly true.)

I'd always been a voracious reader, to the point that my parents had tried to ban me from bringing books to the dinner table at the age of seven, but the depression that had settled over me in LA made it all but impossible to crack the cover of something new or even reread an old favorite. I numbed out in front of TV instead, stuffing down food and eerily feeling like the sitcom studio audiences on-screen were laughing at *me*. As Abilify and circumstances conspired in their alchemic way to make me—against all my own expectations—happier, I found myself desperate to read again, and not just fiction either. I stumbled across Taylor's work not long after *The Body Is Not an Apology* was published, and soon I was seeking out books by adrienne maree brown, Aubrey Gordon, Jes Baker, and other fat-affirming activists—many of whom were members of the LGBTQ+ community themselves, and all of whom rejected the notion that thinness inherently meant worthiness. I sat on the bus or at the diner and turned the pages, fortifying my fatphobic lizard brain with the notion that there was room for all kinds of bodies within the context of queerness; I didn't necessarily believe this truth extended to me, not back then, but at least I was beginning to question the cishet norms I'd unwittingly transplanted onto my new life.

At some point, I started ordering more and more takeout. Sometimes it was in nonbinge capacities, like when I'd get Thai delivery with my roommates and watch movies on Sunday nights, but more often than not, the food was ordered in deliberate excess, especially when a night out hadn't gone the way I wanted. If dating apps ruled my evenings, then food-delivery apps ruled my late nights, and I'd regularly order a whole pizza or a grease-stained mass of mac and cheese or a slew of deep-fried diner appetizers from the Uber Pool on the way home from an unsuccessful first date, the food often reaching my home before I did and growing cold on the stoop by the time I could sneak it upstairs. Most of the time, I ate it anyway, hunched over in bed in front of my laptop, swallowing the warm carbs and savoring the lack of pressure I associated with introducing myself to a new person and nodding and smiling and trying to seem lovable. Alone in my room during a binge, I didn't have to confront the dissonance of harming myself with food even as I consumed the work of writers and artists who made me want to be better, to treat myself better.

When did the pendulum swing to me bingeing regularly again? Was it six months into my time in New York? Nine? A year? I can't be sure, even from studying Caviar and Postmates receipts from that time; the same burrito that would have felt distinctly like a binge at 3:00 a.m. might have taken on a different context if, say, I'd skipped dinner before going out and had no food at home, and I wasn't yet in the habit of keeping a binge log, desperate as I was to reconvince myself that my twice- or thrice-weekly food indiscretions were just this *weird thing I did* (despite all the time I'd put in admitting otherwise at food group back in LA). The memories from that time recede and collapse into themselves, an endless blur of leaving parties drunk and ordering food or purchasing a plastic bag's worth of binge fuel—Pringles, Ben & Jerry's pints, whole jars of jam—at any one of the bodegas that lined my neighborhood's corners.

By the end of my time at *GARAGE*, I was bingeing at least a few times a week, on drunken nights out and stoned, bored nights in alike, and, looking back, I wonder if it was partly *because*, not in spite of, the fact that my life was starting to take shape; I was living in New York, surrounded by friends, doing the kind of work I'd always dreamed of and finally dating the people I'd never dared admit to myself I'd always wanted to date, but—insecure, formerly friendless, perma-dateless loner that I still considered myself to be on some level—I couldn't help waiting for the other shoe to drop.

I didn't trust my own fragile sense of contentment, no matter how hard I knew I'd worked to build it. I feared all the change that was erupting in seemingly every corner of my life, and the version of me who binged at night and woke up early to hide the telltale food bags from her roommates' view at least held some scant illusion of control, something I felt less and less of every time I was handed a new work assignment I didn't know how to execute or got a polite "Let's be friends" text after a date with a girl. I had finally begun putting myself out there—whatever that meant—and now there were stakes to my life, stark and unignorable. I started having a recurring dream of partying on a Brooklyn fire escape, alternately lost in the spontaneity of the moment and pausing to look down and be startled by the dark, vertiginous drop looming below. (My subconscious is rarely subtle.)

I was never more keenly aware of the brand-new stakes my

life had taken on than when I got an email from a *Vogue* editor, toward the end of my first year at *GARAGE*, inviting me to interview for an open culture-writer role on the US Web team. I closed the browser, remembering the *Vogue*s I'd desperately studied in order to prep myself for my current job and feeling like I was going to projectile-vomit the bagel in my stomach (which had been provided courtesy of my then-parent company, as was customary on Friday mornings; years later, when I meet other *Vice* alums, we roll our eyes about the heavy workload and shoddy corporate leadership but still reminisce dreamily about "Bagel Friday").

Once again, I dug my fancy clogs out of my closet and prepared to try to seem impressive. This time, though, I made a stop at the now-closed Bird boutique in Brooklyn before the interview, determined to find a *Vogue*-worthy outfit, even though I knew it was a waste of money to buy something just for an interview. They weren't hiring for a fashion role, and I knew they likely hadn't chosen me for my sartorial acumen, but I still couldn't bring myself to show up at the Condé Nast offices in any of my existing clothes, which suddenly seemed particularly pilly and creatively uninspired.

I left Bird that day with a brand-new pair of Black Crane pants that were one of the only XL-size items I'd been able to find in the whole store. I couldn't remotely afford them, but they were black and loose and cut just innovatively enough to suggest that the person wearing them was extremely cool, in a Brooklyn-artist-who-doesn't-even-care way.

At the last minute, I threw in a belted denim jacket, knowing it would only add to my steadily growing pile of credit card debt but unable to resist the seductive thought of looking like the kind of girl who would (a) own a $200 jean jacket in the first place, and (b) somehow manage not to leave it at a bar. I wore the pants to my first interview and deputized my only other expensive piece of clothing—a black Ali Golden jumpsuit—for the eventual second interview that my would-be manager scheduled for me with none other than *Vogue* editor in chief Anna Wintour, who I was told made a habit of trying to meet most print and Web hires in person before hirings were made official.

In the cab on the way to the interview with Wintour, I vaguely remembered something I'd read about the legendary fashion editor disliking it when interviewees wore black. Too late, I turned to Google, and yep, there it was: a 2017 article in the *Cut* titled "What 10 People Wore to Their Interviews with Anna Wintour" specifically quoted a prospective *Vogue* employee who had splurged on an all-black outfit at Barneys for her interview, only to learn that Wintour allegedly hated black. It wasn't that I was so worried about committing a fashion faux pas—I wasn't a fashion writer, after all, and I sure as hell wasn't a model or influencer—but if this no-black thing was such a known rule, would Wintour or her senior editors think I'd *deliberately* worn the color to be sassy? I definitely planned on pitching provocative ideas for the site if I got the job—in fact, a big reason I was drawn to the idea of leaving my cozy niche at *GARAGE* for *Vogue* was the promise of reaching a wider and more mainstream audience with stories about offbeat pop culture, LGBTQ+ life, and progressive politics that they might not expect even from the online arm of such a storied publication—but the last thing I wanted was to look disrespectful.

Luckily, the all-black thing didn't seem to constitute a nail in my coffin (or maybe my too-expensive jean jacket helped break up the look), because I was offered the culture writer role in the summer of 2019 and started at *Vogue* that September. I cried happy tears when I saw the outpouring of well-wishes from friends and former coworkers that came after I announced my new gig on Twitter, but I was scared to fail, too; accordingly, I binged so badly the night before my first day that I ended up spending the entire next morning bent over the toilet dry-heaving, composing an apologetic email to my new boss in between retches and resolving to never, ever tell anyone that my eating disorder was so out of control that I'd managed to let it rob me of my first day at *Vogue*. (Oops.) When I finally went in the following day, though, I was pleasantly surprised to discover that my new editor Estelle Tang—who'd started at *Vogue* shortly before I had—was so kind and welcoming that I couldn't even muster the requisite energy to feel inadequate; that is, except for the first five minutes of every day when I stepped off the C train and waited for the elevator surrounded by a huddle of my Condé compatriots, the majority of whom were so perfectly groomed and well-heeled even after a sweaty subway ride that I couldn't fathom ever really blending in. I didn't realize back then how much I had in common with many of my new coworkers; it would take joining them in 2019 to help organize what would eventually be called the Condé United campaign to unionize *Vogue*'s parent company for me to see how many experiences we shared, from the difficulty of surviving within an increasingly unstable industry to the all-too-frequent stress created by reporting every morning to what we called "the Content Tower," a company whose publications had helped define the fatphobic, racist, and ableist beauty standards that continued to plague so many of us.

As an editorial assistant at *Teen Vogue* who has written about her own experiences with disordered eating, writer Aiyana Ishmael is all too familiar with the internalized scrutiny and self-doubt that working at an internationally famous media company like Condé Nast can encourage. "*Teen Vogue* is so unique in the magazine landscape for being welcoming and encouraging people to own their differences, so I didn't feel that pressure from the brand itself, but I think I built up the pressure of how I would exist in the rest of the Condé realm," says Ishmael of trying to adjust to the Condé-verse when she first started at *Teen Vogue* in 2021, adding: "It wasn't just struggling with an eating disorder, but also knowing I was probably going to be one of the only fat Black people walking around. I mean, Gabriella [Karefa-Johnson, stylist and *Vogue*'s global fashion director at large until November 2023] is iconic, but I didn't know if she'd actually be in the office."

It's not exactly a secret that the media industry has a long way to go in terms of inclusivity; even in 2023, almost 70 percent of journalists working in the United States are white, and only 10 percent of journalists identify as members of the LGBTQ+ community. Even for those journalists from underrepresented backgrounds who *do* manage to find and maintain full-time employment, circumstances are grim. As I saw firsthand in 2019 through my union work, the low salaries that major media companies paid (and, in many cases, continue to pay) for support staff and entry-level positions often come with a tacit understanding that the people who fill those jobs will have another source of income outside of their work, be it rich parents, a higher-earning partner, or some other way of paying the bills; this leads to an awful lot of media staffers who are (like me) white and from upper-middle-class backgrounds, while workers flung into the box marked "diverse" are forced to decide whether employment at a prestigious brand is worth the sacrifice of trying to survive on what often amounts to less than minimum wage.

It's a lot easier to navigate an intimidating work environment when you have the support of the people around you, even if you weren't initially expecting it. I came into *Vogue* yoked by preconceptions about the people I'd be working with, but organizing alongside them for the better part of three years taught me how fiercely devoted many of them were to building a better and more equitable workplace for ourselves and our colleagues. In retrospect, I think I would have had a much harder time learning to acclimate to life as a not-thin writer at a publication that had historically prized thinness if I hadn't established strong relationships with many of my coworkers early on as a result of our union work; the energy I might have spent bemoaning my lack of thigh gap and resenting my closet's lack of designer clothes was instead spent getting to know my colleagues and asking them what they liked—and didn't like—about their work. When I told the people who became my earliest *Vogue* organizing committee recruits that I loved my job, I wasn't full of it; I did and do, but union organizing taught me that to love something means wanting to see it be the best that it can possibly be, not just accepting it as it's always been.

Of course, you don't have to formally organize a union at your workplace to build solidarity with the people with whom you spend your working hours. Sometimes, just seeing someone who looks like you or shares some major aspect of your identity achieve their goals can inspire you to strive for yours, as Ishmael notes, pointing to the work of former *Vogue* senior fashion and culture editor and current contributor Janelle Okwodu as her own inspiration. "She wrote this story for *Vogue* about being fat and Black and working in the fashion space that I go back to a lot and think was really helpful," continues Ishmael, adding: "Seeing someone higher up and with more experience dealing with so many of these larger issues made me be like 'Okay, I can do this.' For me, I think the biggest thing that helped in getting over my insecurity was just diving in headfirst and owning it, and forcing myself out of my shell even when it's Fashion Week and I go to shows and feel like I'm taking up more than one seat. The person next to you will give you a weird look, like, *This is my seat*, and you're just like, okay, let me try to hold my breath, because maybe that will make me smaller magically."

As I adjusted to my weight gain, one of the first people who made me feel like I could screw up the courage to write about my life as a newly fat person was another *Vogue* contributor: writer, photographer, and plus-size influencer Marielle Elizabeth, who has been writing for the site since 2021 and is the author behind pieces from "Can We Dismantle Fatphobia on the Red Carpet?" to "How to Find the Plus-Size Wedding Dress of Your Dreams." Elizabeth's *Vogue* stories are unafraid to call out anti-fat bias, but they also speak directly to the fat reader, working hard to demystify the "fat experience" (if, indeed, there is such a universal thing) without catering to the gaze of the assumed-thin reader that women's media was long notorious for addressing.

The experience of being one of the few fat people within your workplace can be alienating even in the best of circumstances, and although my current status as a remote employee has meant that I've never actually shared an office with Ishmael or Elizabeth, it brings me deep comfort to see their work pop up online—along with that of Charlotte Zoller, Lydia Okello, Jaelynn Chaney, and many other writers who have contributed to Condé publications on the topic of fatness—and know definitively that I'm not alone, even when my eating disorder is conspiring to make me feel like I am.

When I ask Ishmael how she manages to keep self-doubt—and the disordered-eating mentality it can often trigger—at bay while working in an industry as looks-obsessed and frequently toxic as ours can be, she admits it's not easy. "When I first started [at *Teen Vogue*], it was very easy to get wrapped up in the world of how I wanted to show up and how much space I wanted to take up. In the beginning, it started off easy, and then you have a bad day, which turns into a bad week, and then a bad month, and you feel like you're back at square one, but I'm constantly reminding myself that healing isn't linear," muses Ishmael, adding: "There are going to be good and bad moments where I don't make it to the gym or I decide to eat pizza three nights in a row and I feel like I'm slipping back into old habits and can't control my life, but it doesn't mean that anything about me is wrong. I'm now trying to tell myself that I'm on this journey for the rest of my life, and I'm leaning on the reason I moved to New York and the reason I'm doing the job that I'm doing: it's my purpose, which helps me most days, especially when I'm feeling like 'I shouldn't eat today,' or 'I need to go to the gym twice today.'"

As grateful as I am to be surrounded by colleagues I trust and admire, I'm not immune from succumbing to body anxiety and negative self-talk on those occasions I do go into the Condé Nast headquarters in downtown New York City—which, these days, is a few times a year. The subway commute that used to feel like a slog now strikes me as downright pleasant when I go in to visit, picking up a latte on the way to the 2/3 and listening to boygenius through my headphones on the train platform as I wait to join the scrum of people being whisked off to school or work or wherever they're due in the mornings. (This is one of the nice things I've discovered about remote work; yes, it can get lonely, and yes, I could use a reason to change out of pajamas before 4:00 p.m. every day, but at least now I can appreciate the sheer pleasure of having somewhere to go in New York.)

Despite the novelty of stepping back into my once-daily routine, I still stress about my outfit and my skin and my body— always, my body—on the way into the office when I'm in New York. By the time I actually swipe my ID badge and take the elevator up to the twenty-fifth floor, though, I've usually run into enough of my colleagues that I've forgotten to dwell on my own perceived imperfections; there are shrieks and hugs and exchanges of greetings, there are editors' new babies to inquire after, colleagues' stories to compliment, after-work drinks to mark people's birthdays and last days with, always a plethora of questions to answer in my capacity as a union steward, and frankly, between all that and doing my actual job, I'm too busy to keep up the once-all-consuming work of hating myself full-time. It's a good feeling, one I try not to take for granted.

Although it's taken me a long time and a lot of therapy, I can finally admit that the thing I'm proudest of in my life isn't my job or (occasionally) seeing my byline in print or any other professional accomplishment; it's coming into compassion for the former versions of me, not just the mid-twenties baby dyke and newbie journalist but also the sad girl who sat in her bedroom in LA and ate to quell her loneliness, the deep-closeted college kid, the straight-C high school student and abandoned eighth grader and aughts child of divorce who all still live inside of me, guiding my decisions and shaping my emotional responses. I'm doing my best to heed Joan Didion's famous advice to "keep on nodding terms with the people we used to be, whether we find them attractive company or not." I *don't* find them attractive company, not always, but I'm trying to face them regardless, because I know I can't move forward until I acknowledge the many, many selves who have made me.

Chapter 6

GAIN

When an email titled "U.S. offices working from home," written from Condé Nast's CEO to its entire workforce, hit my inbox on March 12, 2020, I—like so many people who had yet to become familiar with the words "COVID-19," "social distancing," or "PCR test"—was ignorant enough not to be afraid. I pictured a few weeks (two, at most) of sleeping through my commute time, eating lunch that wasn't prepacked in Tupperware, and even spending time with friends. I probably don't have to tell you that none of that ever came to pass, as I spent the next week hunkered down in my apartment with my roommates, leaving only to pick up necessities or occasionally meet Kate and Maya for anxious, six-feet-apart walks in Prospect Park. My friends and I alternately soothed one another and riled up one another's anxieties throughout that strange spring, putting news about what we still called "the coronavirus" into our group chat and distracting ourselves with meaningless celebrity gossip and repetitions of inside jokes that became increasingly less funny as the days wore on.

Soon all my roommates dispersed to go stay with their families until we "had a better sense of what was going on," as we told one another, and soon after that I did the same, only minus the "family" part; my dad was stuck in California, where he'd been teaching for the semester, but his house in Hudson was empty. "Do you really want to be alone up there for God knows how long?" asked my mom worriedly on the phone the night before I rented what felt like the last car at the Hertz on Court Street and found myself driving up the spookily empty Bronx River Parkway, and the truth was, I didn't, but I also didn't want to be alone in my fourth-floor walk-up. My dad's place had space, plenty of light, an outdoor hammock where I could read, an always-stocked kitchen, and at least the vague sense that a real adult was in charge, even if said adult was five thousand miles away. Plus, a family friend in Hudson was out of town and willing to lend me his car; I told myself I'd use it to deliver groceries and do other errands for neighbors, plastering an imagined layer of nobility over my choice to leave the city when, really, I was just scared.

I did deliver groceries in Hudson eventually, meeting up with a mutual aid group my friend Tamar put me in touch with to accept heaving bags of ground meat, fruit, vegetables, and snacks to drop off on doorsteps around town, but what I mostly ended up using the car for during the three or four months I ended up spending alone upstate once then-governor Andrew Cuomo issued a shelter-in-place order in late March was securing binge food (not an easy challenge during that period, when takeout wasn't an option and I didn't leave the house to stock up on provisions more than once every few weeks, but my disordered eating has always loved a challenge; when my mom sent me on the Italian equivalent of an Outward Bound trip the summer after ninth grade—long story—I would set my alarm to wake up in the middle of the night and eat Nesquik with a spoon in the kitchen while everyone else slept).

That spring, I would get in the car and drive to the gas station a few miles from my dad's house whenever I could no longer ignore the seductive mental purr of *Maybe you should binge tonight* that was there to greet me from the moment I woke up, pausing briefly while I worked or went to remote therapy or met up with my friends online for Zoom karaoke—but, ultimately, always reminding me of its presence once night fell. At the gas station, I'd buy bright-red, sharp-cornered boxes of brownie mix and cheap vegetable oil and occasionally even stale eggs if they were in stock, mixing the ingredients in one of my dad's bowls at home before numbing myself on the remaining stash of weed I'd brought up from the city and eating the whole of my uncooked concoction with a mixing spoon in front of the TV in the den. I fell asleep on the couch most nights, unwilling to grant myself the gift of clean sheets and a warm duvet; I'd wake up dry-throated and damp-eyed in the middle of the night, occasionally moving myself to my bedroom but sometimes staring out at the crisp slice of moon I could see out the window for hours, nausea roiling in my belly and making me unable to fall back asleep.

Maybe it's strange that I never consciously shopped for my binges on my biweekly trips to the ShopRite in town, but that's never been how it's worked for me; to plan a binge would be to take the essential motor out of it, to attempt to impose some measure of prior knowledge or control over an act that feels so declaratively *out* of control (except when I'm in the middle of a binge, a time when I often feel strangely powerful, to the extent that I allow myself to feel anything at all; here it is, the bad thing, the thing I spend so much of my time trying to avoid and swear each time I'll never do again; to actually enact it feels almost like a sad kind of freedom).

At first, I filled my grocery-store cart with the same kind of Weight Watchers–approved staples I'd bought ever since I'd reactivated my membership in the diet program when I moved back to Brooklyn—kale; skim milk; avocados; boneless, skinless chicken breasts—but as the weeks wore on and my mental health dipped accordingly (not an uncommon experience during quarantine, a time when global rates of anxiety and depression skyrocketed by 25 percent), I began to temporarily suspend most of my food rules, realizing I couldn't rely on my usual food strategy of shopping virtuously and then ordering takeout to fill myself with all the cheese and carbs and sweets I really craved. This was in the short-lived yet intense era when people were hoarding toilet paper and cleaning supermarkets out of bags of flour, and for the first time in my privileged US-millennial life, I couldn't trust the supermarket to have in stock whatever I was (or wasn't) allowing myself to eat; I felt trapped, and, predictably enough, I craved the heavy, fattening foods I knew would help smother that feeling.

After about a month or so of quarantine, I began to fill my days scrolling *Bon Appétit* and the *New York Times* recipe pages for cooking ideas, meticulously planning my grocery lists and allowing myself to make pretty much whatever I wanted—regardless of caloric content—for maybe the first time ever. I'd cooked before, and I'd certainly indulged at meals before, but unless I was preparing pasta for a dinner party or cookies to bring to a work potluck, I never used butter or white bread or Parmesan or any of the carbs or high-fat dairy items I associated with the dishes I craved the most. (Today, every time I cook a truly satisfying meal, I send a silent message to my younger self across space and time: *One day, you will cook with butter, and it won't feel like such a big deal.*)

The meals I made in Brooklyn once or twice a week were selected primarily for their packed-lunch potential, so I wouldn't have to spend a small daily fortune on a sandwich and a side in the Condé cafeteria (something I often ended up doing anyway, my leftovers forgotten in the office fridge until my weekly Friday clean-out). I'd never cooked with such abandon, and I tried to let that newfound creative license compensate for all the social interaction I wasn't getting, telling myself that it was okay that I didn't know when I'd see my friends or family again, because hey, look at me, I was making tahini brownies and nightly pitchers of margaritas and messaging girls I couldn't actually meet up with on dating apps and organizing *Sex and the City* table reads for my friends on Zoom! Wasn't I having a good time, making a go of it despite my solitude, just like I had for so much of my life? (Intellectually, I understood that many people were as alone as I was, and that aloneness wasn't a reflection on any of us, but the friendless eighth grader who still seemed to rule a part of my brain still associated loneliness with rejection.)

During those months in Hudson, I made ricotta gnocchi and vegan cashew-dill dip and Dutch baby pancakes and even attempted my own version of my beloved Xi'an Famous Foods spicy cumin lamb noodles, always posting an artfully arranged bowl of the finished product on Instagram. I was so culinarily prolific, in fact, that Julie—one of Eliza's and my mutual friends from LA—noted admiringly to Eliza on the phone that it seemed like I was "doing really well." I laughed when Eliza relayed that message, but a little bitterly, knowing that what I *didn't* post on Instagram was my brownie-mix drives, my strings of nights spent staring vacantly at the TV, my stoned binges on leftovers from the hearty meals I'd cooked (which always felt like the ultimate sin, somehow; I'd made those meals with the best of intentions, trusting my future self to *just be cool*, and now my present self had betrayed that trust).

I don't know exactly how I would have looked back at this period of my life, food-wise, if it hadn't coincided with the very first scarlet stretch marks cracking the previously smooth skin of my stomach. There were two of them one day in April, as boldly etched as though I'd given them permission to be there, and then one morning a week or two later, there were more. I didn't know if the weight gain they signified (which I was too afraid to confirm by stepping on my dad's scale but could gauge from how my jeans fit on the rare occasion I changed out of sweatpants) came from bingeing or putting Weight Watchers on pause during quarantine or some combination thereof, but I tried vaguely to make the best of it, ordering a plethora of new clothes online when my best pair of jeans ceased to fit and my T-shirts began sitting disarmingly tight on my chest (a style I'd learned to eschew when I developed early and suddenly realized—in the way twelve-year-old girls are so often forced to—that anything other than a loose fit would all but guarantee catcalls).

I spent so much of the money I was lucky to still be earning in quarantine on clothes, from essentials like bras that I genuinely needed to replace (in theory, at least, given that nobody was actually seeing me from the neck down) to branded items from New York restaurants I loved that had been hit hard by the pandemic to—mostly—stupid shit I didn't need, like a pink faux-fur-trimmed tank top I bought primarily because Jazmine had one, too. I shopped because I had nothing to do, because everyone I normally turned to for support was having as hard a time as I was (if not more so), because I didn't feel like I had the right to my sadness when so many people were losing their health and jobs and homes and even their loved ones, because my hunger wouldn't cease and my body was getting bigger and when I was moving a pair of limited-edition Phoebe Bridgers merch sweatpants to my cart and clicking Purchase, I didn't have to think about any of it.

I haven't weighed myself consistently since the most disordered days of my dieting obsession in LA, but I would estimate that I gained about forty pounds in the first year of the pandemic, on top of the thirty or so pounds that had settled on my frame in New York after over a year of furtive bingeing, and I quickly repledged fealty to Weight Watchers the next morning. During my time at *GARAGE*, I'd started to care a little bit more about what I wore on any given day, an interest that dovetailed with the end of my ability to fit into the straight sizes offered by most of the low-femme-basics stores I shopped at, like Madewell and Urban Outfitters; eventually, though, Maya clued me in to the offerings of Universal Standard, a size-inclusive brand out of New York that runs from 00–40 and designates its 14–16 offering as a "Small." I'd accrued some dressy staples from there, including a pair of butter-soft turtlenecks and a long, silky, ink-black dress whose hem swished the floor, and those still fit me after my quarantine weight gain, but pretty much nothing else did.

Like so many other people who were remotely employed during the first outbreak of COVID-19 in the States, I wasn't leaving the house on any kind of regular basis until June 2020, and until then, I didn't see the shape of my new body reflected back to me by the eyes of the world. I caught glimpses of myself in mirrors, though, noting the sudden prominence of my double chin or the waggle of the flesh under my upper arms; I tried not to receive these sights with hatred, but I wasn't always successful, and when I reached a particular point of despair over my shifting form, food was always there to soothe me. Binge eating and weight gain became linked in a way they hadn't really been before, when I was still in the habit of restricting in the aftermath of my binges and exercising regularly; even in Brooklyn, I'd half-heartedly used the elliptical at the Crunch near me and gone on weekly, huffing-and-puffing runs in Prospect Park, but I moved less during the initial quarantine phase of the pandemic than I ever had, and the emotional bonds that tethered me to food were as strong and starkly defined as they ever had been before.

I'd left Brooklyn for Hudson on the precipice of what I considered to be "fat" at the time (admittedly, a moving target, given that I'd also thought I was fat when I was barely heavy enough to menstruate regularly in LA) and returned at the start of that summer significantly outside of what the scary, bold-typed graph I'd looked up on the internet determined to be my "healthy weight." For months, I'd been squeezing myself into the size L gym shorts I'd bought in packs of three at the Target on Atlantic when I first moved into the Prospect Heights apartment, but by June 2020, I could barely fit into an XL; a 2XL fit tightly around my hips for the first time ever, and while my body weight had been fluctuating since roughly the age of fourteen, this was the largest I'd ever seen myself. I wasn't happy about it—far from it, in fact—but in retrospect, I think writing about the experience professionally helped me find language (and, thus, control) around the terror of fatness that I'd so long held within myself; I couldn't keep up the energy that detesting my physical form required if I was also tasked with writing about it on a regular basis.

It was around the pandemic that I began covering what I called "the body beat" at *Vogue*, first reporting out a piece in March 2020 about how people living with eating disorders were faring under lockdown. (In case you were wondering, the answer was: not well, unsurprisingly. "Eating disorders creep up when you're isolated, or anxious, or under the weather. They thrive in these conditions," one expert I spoke to for that story told me, and accordingly, I don't know anyone living with an eating disorder who didn't experience at least *some* spike in ED mentality during those terrifying first few months of the pandemic.) Eight months later, I published a personal essay about the difficulty I had not eating compulsively during the winter holidays, naming myself publicly as someone who lived with binge eating disorder for the first time, and once the first COVID-19 vaccines became available, I wrote a story about BMI being qualified as a comorbidity that entitled many people with obesity (including myself) to an early jab.

Published in February 2021 and titled "Millions of Americans Qualify for the COVID-19 Vaccine Based on BMI. Why Should We Apologize for It?," that last story situated me squarely within the large demographic of fat people who regularly had their personal responsibility and dignity called into question by a BMI-worshipping medical establishment; I identified myself as fat right in the lede, and while there were things about the story I would change if I were writing it now, I ended on what I still hope is a galvanizing note: "Do I have anxieties, fears, and reservations about letting my BMI determine my vaccine eligibility? Sure, but I didn't make the rules—New York State did—and I value my personal health, both physical and mental, enough to accept protection from COVID-19 despite the inner voice that tells me that, as a fat person, I don't deserve it." The BMI piece, which owed much to what I'd recently learned from reading *Fearing the Black Body*, provoked more of a response than anything else I'd ever written, to the point where I recorded a guest spot on NPR's *All Things Considered* to discuss it—and, after the spot aired, ended up the humble recipient of a torrent of unasked-for opinions about everything from my downright *dangerous* fat acceptance to the vocal fry that one man claimed was endemic to "young women of your generation."

I was embarrassed when I read the unsolicited emails from these people I didn't know, just like I was when I then finally listened to myself on the show and mentally supplied what I wished I'd said for what I'd actually said. Still, maybe it was a sign of progress that I also thought: *Fuck you.* I was proud of the story; if some men were mad that I sounded like a fat-affirming millennial woman when discussing it, well, I *was* a fat-affirming millennial woman, and they could choke. (Ultimately, though, even the mostly positive reaction to that story made me feel vaguely like a fraud, as I almost always did when I wrote stories that fell under the broad rubric of "body positivity"—I don't undervalue the significance of getting to publish specifically fat-positive content at an institution like *Vogue*, but I also don't delude myself about the potential of that content to single-handedly fix the severe systemic problems that ail the still-fatphobic fashion and media industries.)

As I did more research about how people who were already predisposed to struggle with food and weight were faring during the pandemic, I came across plenty of reassurance that I was far from the only one whose physical form looked different in the winter of 2021 than it had during the spring of 2020. Author, lecturer, and weight-based discrimination expert Virgie Tovar, who has written extensively about both the individual and systemic experiences of living in a fat body, recently summarized the situation to me thus: "In times of stress or fear, people focus more than usual on the things that they believe they can control. This is called terror management or threat management. If we look at the data, we actually don't have a lot of control over our body size long-term (meaning that if you're naturally a larger person, you will likely always be a larger person or if you're naturally a smaller person, you will likely always be a smaller person), but our culture teaches us that we have complete control over it. Our culture also teaches us that gaining weight is a sign of moral failure and ugliness. So you take all of that, mix it up, and you've got this fraught cocktail that we saw come together during the pandemic."

It was a potent cocktail indeed, one whose intoxicating effect was ramped up all the more by the weird, frozen-in-time quality of the early pandemic. Eliza was just a half-hour drive away from me, quarantining with her boyfriend, Zack, and their new puppy, Elvis, but I rarely let myself see them even outside, sure that if any of us got sick, it would somehow be my fault. The first time we dared to hang out indoors in late May, I sat on Eliza's couch with Elvis's velvet-soft ears between my fingers like rosary beads and began sobbing from some guttural place inside me, responding to her worried reaction through tears: "What if the world never goes back to normal, and I'm single forever?" It sounds humiliatingly trivial now, like the complaint a stock rom-com heroine would have if she improbably found herself living through a global pandemic, but I'd only just begun to date the people I actually wanted to date; I couldn't stand the thought of spending the rest of my twenties—the "fun years" everyone had promised were on the horizon when I'd been a miserable, lonely teen—in lockdown, a possibility that no scientist or doctor was totally willing to rule out back in the days when we were still wiping down our groceries with Clorox.

It wasn't that I'd been having so much fun dating in New York; a big breakup with the first woman I'd had a real emotional connection with had sidelined me just a few weeks into my time at *Vogue*, and in its aftermath, I'd fallen right back into my pattern of exhaustive thrice-weekly first dates followed by compensatory binges. During quarantine, though, my prosaic desperation about my newly enlarged body melded with my far-from-unique concerns about COVID, all this anxiety amounting to very little time that *wasn't* spent going over one or another in a litany of fears. I was terrified both that I'd be cut off from society forever and—perhaps even more darkly— that I'd have to reenter the world and try to find love at my current weight; every day that I woke up fat and did my best to care for myself felt like a quiet personal revolution, but I still wasn't secure enough to imagine that there might be a potential partner out there who would truly love a body over which I finally seemed to have lost control. "Before you love anyone else, you have to love yourself," goes the old cliché, but I'd been doing my best to love myself (or at least like myself) for years; at what point would it stop feeling like work?

I eventually returned to a life that approximated normal back in Brooklyn, especially once vaccines were released and it began to seem less morally suspect to gather a few friends indoors for dinner or even go to a movie masked. I still worked remotely, but my roommates were all home during the day, too, and with the four of us regularly convening over meals and co-working in the living room, it was harder to disappear behind the scrim of loneliness that had accompanied the blow of my quarantine weight gain. I still paid the depressing sum of $20 a month for Weight Watchers, but I went off it all the time, resetting my weekly points daily and resenting my active monetary participation in diet culture even as I clung to its semblance of imposed order like a buoy in shifting seas.

I talked about all of this—my meta-shame over paying for Weight Watchers, my stress over my weight gain, my discomfort at suddenly being confronted with the kind of societal fatphobia I'd always known existed but, frankly, hadn't cared to investigate all that much when I was thin—in my weekly session with Emily, the therapist I'd started seeing a few months after I'd started at *Vogue* and with the circle of fat and fat-positive friends I'd begun to cultivate since moving to New York, exulting in the feeling of being understood even when I didn't quite understand myself. The same *Fuck you* that had echoed in my head after reading the criticism of my NPR spot suddenly appeared when I read a fatphobic feature from a major news outlet, or saw a fat-shaming online account retweet one of my "body beat" stories, or endured a not-so-subtle familial inquiry about my weight. I tapped into the anger by getting tattoos, one on each forearm and a smaller one on the curve of my right thigh, gleefully staking claim to a body that—despite its new size—never felt more like mine than when someone slowly and painfully inked a design I'd chosen into its skin.

Slowly, as I resumed spending weekend nights with Kate and Maya, getting dinner with Jazmine and her now-fiancé Gabe, and even dating again—albeit with a slightly less manic energy than I'd brought to the proceedings prior to the pandemic—I even began to feel some compassion for the version of me that had existed in quarantine. Yes, I'd binged, but I'd also cooked and shopped and driven and worked and gone to therapy and done my best to be there for my neighbors and loved ones and even headed out for some slow, halting runs down the road leading toward my dad's house; didn't all those things count? I tried to remind myself that there was value in all of it, despite the bingeing and whether I'd "gotten fat" or not (this was the body-shaming vernacular I still reached for then, evaluating myself with the passive cruelty of a bitchy neighbor gossiping over bad wine). For the first time, though, I started to temper the shame of bingeing with uncharacteristic ease on myself the day after a binge, remaking my bed with clean sheets and rehydrating with room-temperature water and allowing my body to take the time it needed to recover from what I was still doing to it on a regular basis.

"I think COVID-19 gave me new respect for my body. I got to watch my body take on such a massive amount of stress and still manage to get out of bed and work through a really scary experience by laughing, crying, dancing, stomping, sleeping, having sex, writing, drawing, and cooking," reflects Tovar, but sadly, this narrative isn't one I've heard a lot of people express about how they got through the early days of COVID. "Quarantine fifteen" jokes were everywhere back then, as though the worst possible thing that could befall you during a deadly global pandemic was gaining a little extra cushioning around your thighs and belly. (I resented the hell out of these jokes, especially when they were made by thin people, but I couldn't help relating to them anyway; after all, wasn't I still wrestling with the bodily insecurity that my quarantine-induced weight gain had brought on? Was the only difference between me and the skinny women posting fatphobic quarantine memes on my Instagram feed the fact that I was now . . . actually fat?)

A National Institutes of Health study about COVID-19 and weight gain published in January 2022 polled more than three thousand individuals about how their bodies had changed throughout the pandemic, finding that 48 percent had gained weight—and that within the category of people who reported being very overweight before the pandemic, that number jumped to 65 percent. As of 2021, 78 percent of people hospitalized with COVID-19 were overweight or had obesity, but the mainstream-media narrative that began to emerge wasn't about how practitioners could sensitively and responsibly treat those patients, or even about how those patients could best advocate for themselves within an expressly fatphobic health-care system; instead, scare-mongering stories about the personal and public-health imperative to lose weight abounded, with perhaps the worst of them being a 2021 *New York Times* article titled "The Pandemic as a Wake-Up Call for Personal Health."

In the piece, Jane E. Brody—the author of the article and *Times*'s designated Personal Health columnist—took Americans to task for all that oh-so-calorically-unacceptable bread-baking that many of us with the luxury of time and remote jobs had done during quarantine, writing sniffily: "While I understood their need to relieve stress, feel productive and perhaps help others less able or so inclined, bread, muffins and cookies were not the most wholesome products that might have emerged from pandemic kitchens." I listened for the *Fuck you* in my head when I read that sentence, and it came instantly, but I noticed it was accompanied by a little twist of what I just barely recognized as shame. Why *had* I been such a pig, eaten so much, baked in good moods and binged in bad moods and focused my energy on keeping myself afloat instead of committing to a diet-and-exercise plan that would have left me toned and slim by the time it was safe to rejoin the outside world?

Luckily, I've had enough therapy and exposure to fat-positive rhetoric at this point to be able to note decisively that Brody's personal food choices (which she goes on to detail at length in the article, proudly noting that she's most definitely "not a fanatic when it comes to food" due to the presence of "cookies, crackers and even chips in my cupboard") aren't particularly relevant to my life or to the lives of any other fat people, whether they gained weight during COVID or have been fat their whole lives or—like me—saw their bodies change slowly and then suddenly thanks to the evolution of an underlying eating disorder. My bingeing habits may have ramped up during quarantine, but they were hardly new to me; what *was* new was dispensing with Weight Watchers—albeit temporarily—and giving myself a license to eat whatever I wanted in nonbinge contexts. I still think the bingeing was most directly responsible for my weight gain, not the no-knead bread that I made (ironically, from a *New York Times* recipe) during one of the hardest and most isolated periods that I and many people I know have ever lived through—but if it *had* been the bread, would that have been so bad?

I've been thin and I've been fat, and one of the most stark differences between the former category and the latter is the way that some thin people seem to assume that being fat makes you . . . if not dumb, well, at least a little less smart than *they* are. After all, why would you bake sugary cakes to ballast yourself throughout the stress and loneliness of a global pandemic if you *really* understood what you were doing to yourself? Why *wouldn't* an equally intelligent person just willpower their way down to what the graph I'd looked up online at the end of quarantine referred to as a "healthy weight"? (As though it were that simple, as though it were their business.) Articles like Brody's perform the dismal magic trick of turning fat bodies into community property to be spoken about, but never *to*; the barely obscured supposition is that fatness isn't a bodily state or—God forbid—an identity, but a moral failing, a problem to be solved by any means necessary.

I remember enjoying the Sociology of Food seminar I took my senior year of college, in which my professor talked to us about the structural barriers to fresh food, time off, and safe outdoor space that caused or contributed to many Americans' struggles with obesity, but I never truly confronted the idea of fatness as anything other than the health issue/aesthetic eyesore/moral failing that society loves to present it as until I (a) became fat myself, and (b) read Kate Harding and Marianne Kirby's 2009 book *Lessons from the Fat-o-sphere* in the middle of the second year of the pandemic, a time when I felt stuck somewhere between fat acceptance (for other people) and internalized fatphobia (for me). "If you are dead-set on hating yourself, this isn't the book for you," wrote one reviewer on the used-book site where I'd purchased my copy, and the note filled me with some trepidation, but even more curiosity. What would I do—who would I be?—without my self-hatred?

With its scarlet cover and bold typeface, *Lessons from the Fat-o-sphere* announces the second it's in your possession that it's not one of those diet-culture-endorsed tomes that appropriate the rhetoric of wellness/self-care culture in trying to convince you that losing weight is always the best choice "for *you*"; the book is as clear a repudiation as I've ever read of that kind of thinking, linking fatphobia to deeply entrenched systems of sexism, racism, anti-Blackness, and anti-LGBTQ+ sentiment that are impossible to uproot or disrupt by hyper-focusing on the size of one's own body. (The idea of dieting as distraction, rather than discipline, was new to me, but it made sense; it's very hard to do anything, let alone organize to make systemic change in your community or workplace, when you're fucking starving.) Diet culture, and the lifelong obsession with thinness that it planted in me, had me at war with myself for the first two and a half decades of my life, but the subtitle of Harding and Kirby's book encouraged the reader to "declare a truce with your body," something I hadn't even realized I needed permission for until I encountered it in literary form.

One of the narratives from *Lessons from the Fat-o-sphere* that jarred me the most was the essay written by a woman whose mother had died of a preventable disease after her doctor had sent her home from an appointment, telling her not to come back until she'd lost fifty pounds. Reflecting on the story, I suddenly realized I hadn't seen a doctor since well before the pandemic, even though my Condé insurance would have covered the cost of a physical. I told myself I'd been busy, that it hadn't been safe at first to go to a doctor for nonemergency care, and those things were true, but equally true was the fact that I didn't want to step on a scale in a paper gown with my ass exposed and hear from a doctor just how much damage I'd done to myself. I was one of the privileged few in digital media who actually had access to the comprehensive health insurance a staff job affords, yet I'd let shame and internalized self-loathing rob me of taking advantage of it. (There is so much that fatphobia stands ready and waiting to take from us if we don't receive the support we need to fight back against it; I still grieve the things I lost to its insidious presence in my life, even as I refuse to give up even more.)

Reading *Lessons from the Fat-o-sphere* cracked something open inside me, and soon I was following more and more fat and proudly fat-positive writers, artists, activists, and influencers on Instagram and Twitter, from Tovar herself to Roxane Gay to Aubrey Gordon to S. Bear Bergman. I exulted in their crop-top photos and their business attire (especially when they were one and the same), their carefully researched essays and their haphazardly composed Notes-app poems, their home-cooked meals and their on-the-fly takeout on road trips, taking each image and caption I saw as evidence that the size of my body didn't have to disqualify me from living the kind of big, bold life I'd once thought only dieting could give me. Every time I saw a fat person loving and being loved out loud on the internet, it felt like some immeasurable unit of the hatred I had for my new body dissolved, and I even began to see myself as a tiny part of that lineage, reading and rereading grateful emails and DMs from fat readers who'd felt seen by my *Vogue* stories and allowing myself to feel momentarily proud instead of reflexively false and instantly nauseous.

I wish *Lessons from the Fat-o-sphere* and I had crossed paths earlier, back when I was still thin, so I could have learned how to challenge at least some of my fatphobic preconceptions before they were explicitly relevant to my body and life (much in the same way I wish that I'd sought out or been taught literally anything meaningful about LGBTQ+ history before I came out at twenty-five). That's not how it worked out, though, and these days, I try to content myself with being a voice from the other side—the fat side, the unapologetic side, the "stared down the scarlet F and turned out okay" side—for people who I know or sense are struggling with the same kind of toxic push-pull around body size and self-worth that I grappled with for years. Being fat didn't cure me of my internalized fatphobia or permanently dispel any unease I had around living in a larger body, but it did force me to confront a living reality I'd spent multiple decades fearing; I'm not saying everybody out there needs to gain weight in order to confront their demons, but I do think pretty much everyone could benefit from accepting the fact that gaining weight is not, in and of itself, a universally negative thing.

Today, I can honestly say I wouldn't trade anything in my life to be thin again, but I ache for the lost years when that wasn't true, when I would have given anything I had and then some for a visible rib cage. Back then, I could scarcely imagine that one day I'd be an out, queer, fat writer doing the kind of work I cared about, and I know a younger me might have seen my present-day weight as a failure, but I'm now firmly invested in pushing back against that kind of thinking—in my own mind, and in the minds of the people around me, too, many of whom are starting to see their physical forms change as they grow into full-fledged adults, adults whose bodies work and age and grow tomatoes in the dirt and take up weight lifting and house babies and get gender-affirming surgery and quit barre class and generally undergo the evolution associated with what the luckiest among us get to call life.

"I spent so much of my life living in absolute sheer terror of gaining weight because I was told—and I believed—that being fat was the worst thing that could ever happen to me. It turns out, nothing was further from the truth. Deciding to accept and love my fat body has brought me on a wildly gorgeous adventure that truly wasn't available to me before," says Tovar, adding, "When I finally accepted that I was always going to be fat, I felt joy and relief (because to me that meant I could stop dieting and stop hating my body), but also grief and loss (I had spent twenty years trying to achieve this 'dream life' I believed would come once I became thin and I had to let go of all that and begin to build a new dream). It takes a long time to put blame where it belongs—on a culture that promotes overtly negative beliefs and attitudes about a group of people and the individuals who adopt those beliefs and attitudes—not on yourself. Remember: it's never your fault that we live in a fat-hating culture."

As Tovar notes, rejecting the insidious fatphobia spoon-fed to us by so much of the dominant culture isn't a quick, easy, or painless process, but—having initiated it sometime in the aftermath of quarantine, less with one decisive action than with a constellation of small choices about how I wanted to live my life—I can attest that it's been far more rewarding and meaningful than the much longer chunk of time and energy I devoted to trying to make (and keep) myself as small as possible. Do I still have insecurities about my body? Of course, but I'm more realistic about anticipating those insecurities and giving myself the mental "you are valid at any size" lectures necessary to dispel them; and when I can't muster up the lecture myself, I can count on my therapist or my partner or one of my closest friends to give it to me, which would have meant the world to the whippet-thin, deeply lonely version of me who ate to temporarily still her craving for community in all its forms.

"Loving and protecting my fat body is why I'm my own boss, why I have a thriving business, why I learned to set boundaries with people, why I stopped dating jerks, why I get to travel the world, write books, teach corporate clients how to create accessible work spaces, why I have amazing friends, why I have a partner who worships my body, why I have a fire in my belly, why I'm no-contact with my toxic family, why every item of clothing in my closet makes me feel amazing, why I reconnected to my intuition, why I'm able to advocate for better sex, why I

always know I have a purpose," kvells Tovar, and while I sometimes struggle to appreciate all that's happened in my life since
I slowly began to accept my fat body as a direct consequence of
that acceptance, I know on a deeper level that none of it would
have happened without the other fat people who pointed me in
the right direction when I was first struggling to deal with my
weight gain.

All too often, the role of the "influencer" is scoffed at (perhaps in part because of the portal to fame and power it can
provide to traditionally marginalized creators), but the fat influencers and artists and writers and actors and musicians I sought
out on social media when I first began to exceed the sizes that
most stores kept in stock (or even manufactured) provided the
road map that pointed me toward my current identity as a fat,
mostly happy, out-and-proud dyke and decidedly fat-positive
human being. At twenty-nine, I'm aware that my body may hold
infinitely more change within it (*baruch hashem*), but one thing I
refuse to let go of—whether I stay my current size the rest of my
life, lose weight, gain weight, or any combination thereof—is the
hard-won knowledge that none of its permutations could ever
really be wrong.

Chapter 7

MOVE

If I had to estimate, I would say I've gone on about three hundred runs over the past six or seven years, lacing up my sneakers and trudging out my front door in everything from the dry LA heat to the Brooklyn winter cold to the sweaty gray mist that seems to envelop much of Austin, Texas—the city I left Brooklyn for in September 2021—after the rainy season passes.

That number surprises me even now, but I suppose it encompasses a lot of time, time when I've dutifully headed out every day for a week and, alternately, let my running shoes and fanny pack gather dust in the corner of my bedroom while I go on a days-long binge. As I write this, I realize I haven't logged into my Nike Run Club app in months—these days, I get most of my cardio in by swimming laps at the free public pool near my apartment, or running on the elliptical while I mainline *The Real Housewives of New Jersey* on the gym TV—

but running was the first form of exercise that ever really lit me up inside, and I don't think I would have found my way to my current, stable, sometimes-even-joyful relationship with exercise without it.

I don't think of running as a particularly malleable discipline, but when I bought a pair of Pumas half-off at a TV prop sale in LA and headed out for my first meandering run on the dirt path behind my office—wincing between strides when I heard my unstretched knees crack audibly but eventually exulting in the weightless feeling of sprinting downhill I unknowingly initiated a long-term relationship with the sport, one that would grow, fluctuate, and transform itself many times over. Over the years, running has by turns occupied the foreground of my life and receded far into the background, and though my relationship with it has definitely suffered as a result of my disordered eating, I can't deny the power it's brought me to know I can rely on myself and my body for the duration of a twenty-four-minute run. (That's how long I've always run for: twenty-four minutes exactly, no more, no less, always timed to the beat of the playlists I rely on to propel me through the park or around the trail or between the stoplights dotting the sidewalks of whatever city I'm in.)

I've gone on some runs for the sheer purpose of burning calories, trying to make it a mile and a half straight without stopping or passing out from the sheer lack of food in my stomach, and I've gone on others that were slow and sweet and gentle on my hips and calves and ankles, waving at other runners on the path ahead of me and letting the clean air wash over me while the sun dipped lower and lower in the sky. Most of the time, though, embarking on a run is a medium-level chore at best, even on the rare occasions when I'm stringing several runs together per week and shaving seconds—if not minutes—off my mile time with each one. I never, ever want to go; I always dread the finding of my sneakers and the wedging on of one of my dozen somehow-always-too-small sports bras and the cramp that reliably makes my calves ache when I first set out, but when I've gone on runs over the past three or four years, it's almost always been because I know how good I'll feel *after* (especially if I've eaten enough beforehand to keep my blood sugar from dipping).

That wasn't always the case, though, least of all when I was twenty-four and still living in LA. When I first began regularly running around the length of the Silver Lake Reservoir in 2017, I was doing it less for the intrinsic joy of movement and more for the promise of thinness that the activity represented. Running wasn't the first or only form of exercise I employed in service of that goal, but the spin classes I favored for their ability to pack maximum caloric offset into a forty-five-minute session were too expensive for me to attend regularly, and the pulled-together waifishness of seemingly every other woman at the barre class I'd reluctantly checked out on a coworker's recommendation dissuaded me from ever going back (as if the visual comparison weren't enough, the barre class itself made my thighs and fore-arms shake uncontrollably as I attempted to control muscles I wasn't actually sure I possessed). Running was free, it was almost always available, and—most important to me, back then—it was at least enough exercise to underwrite as much milk in my coffee as I wanted.

When I moved back to New York and started Abilify, though, my relationship with running began to change. The charm of unyielding blue sky and view of the empty reservoir I'd gotten used to having as my backdrop while I ran in LA had gotten absorbed in the fog of my depression relatively quickly, but the loop of Prospect Park I completed once or twice a week was verdant and bustling in summer, ice-frosted and pleasantly silent in winter, golden-leaved and somehow cider-scented in fall, and, best of all, perfectly crisp and bracing in spring, particularly in those first few months of March and April when the air was newly warm enough to run without a sweatshirt. There were other runners I got used to seeing as we set off on our paths, and though it's been a few years since I ran in that particular park, I remember them even now; the young mom with the jogging stroller, the guy who ran in shorts no matter the season, and—my favorite—the sweet-faced elder dyke in the Provincetown sweatshirt who sometimes walked the loop with a gray-haired friend or lover.

In the very worst of the heat and cold that New York had to offer, I resigned myself to using the elliptical at Crunch, but even that felt less punitive than my sporadic gym workouts had in LA. I had always detested the routine of remembering to pack a gym bag, schlepping it to work, and then hauling its contents into an invariably sweaty and crowded locker room, but the ride from my office in the Financial District to the Crunch on Flatbush Ave required me to transfer to the Q train, which Maya had taught me to treasure for its aboveground route; I would almost always get a seat, and I'd stare out the opposite window and watch the city fly by me, jewel-like and flickering, while I psyched myself up with one of the dozens of running playlists I'd started to put together for myself on Spotify (a perusal of which reveals a whole lot of SOPHIE, Charli XCX, Hannah Diamond, and other hyperpop and PC Music artists delivering dry lyrics over a frenetic beat).

When I first rented the 2019 comedy *Brittany Runs a Marathon* during quarantine, I was excited to see a portrayal of a fat runner that didn't seem to be implicitly steeped in ridicule. I liked the star, Jillian Bell, and although I was secretly uneasy about the fact that the few runs I was still forcing myself to go on weren't helping me lose weight (in fact, the number on the scale in the bathroom seemed to be going up by the month), I was at least putatively over enough of my internalized fatphobia and self-loathing by then to recognize that I *shouldn't* be worried about it. At first, I felt delightfully seen by Bell's character Brittany, an insecure, seemingly forever-wingwoman who partied hard and slept late and tried to scam her doctor into prescribing her Adderall while tugging her sleeves down to obscure the fresh club stamps on her hands; as I watched Brittany take up running and start to lose weight, though, drawing compliments from the world as the actress portraying her gradually had her fat suit depadded, I heard an old and—I'd thought—long-defeated voice pipe up in the back of my mind: Was *that* what was supposed to happen to me? Why was I committing to running at all if it wasn't going to help me be thin—and, really, should I even bother?

Intellectually, I understood that the movie wasn't telling the audience that it was 100 percent *good* that Brittany had lost weight—in fact, the script telegraphed pretty clearly that Brittany's weight loss lined up directly with her increased vanity and selfishness—but still, I couldn't help wishing that Brittany had simply . . . stayed the size she was at the start of the film, as so many people do in spite of discovering new physical activities and nurturing a passion for physical movement in adulthood. I loved where the film left Brittany—still running, albeit less obsessively, and finally dating Jern, the sweet, couch-surfing weirdo she'd originally fallen for when she was too closed-off and full of self-loathing to make a relationship work—but it would have meant a lot more to me to watch a still-fat Brittany tell off her toxic roommate, get a clean(er) bill of health from her doctor, take the leap of loving and being loved by Jern, and, yes, run the New York Marathon, if only to demonstrate that all these wonderful changes *could still have happened if she hadn't lost the weight.*

I wasn't the only one who was disappointed by the emphasis that *Brittany Runs a Marathon* placed on weight loss for its own sake. In a 2019 *Vulture* article titled "Brittany Didn't Need to Lose Weight to Run a Marathon," writer Madison Malone Kircher points to the existence of a large and diverse community of fat runners who do not practice the sport with the primary goal of losing weight: "In *Brittany Runs a Marathon*, being fat is portrayed as a starting point instead of just a state of being. Brittany getting her life in order is inextricably linked to her weight loss." It's this same all-too-common framework of "fat as starting point" that's always held me back from thinking of myself as a "real" runner, even during the periods of my life when I averaged ten to fifteen miles a week. I told myself I didn't want to seem braggy, knowing how much it annoyed me when other people (especially people thinner than I was) wouldn't shut up about their workouts, but really, I still saw myself as the shy third grader who made daisy chains on the outfield while everyone else played softball—I'd never been anything resembling an athlete, and gaining weight sure as hell didn't help me feel like one.

Ultimately, the part of *Brittany Runs a Marathon* that made me tear up alone in front of my laptop wasn't the weight loss; it was the recognition I felt when Brittany accepted shitty treatment from her gang of basic-hot-girl "going out" friends, when she let herself flirt with a guy only to be crudely propositioned for a blow job seconds after, when she continually cut herself down and closed herself off from the world because she didn't believe she deserved to fully participate in it at her size (which, it should be said, appeared to be roughly that of the average American woman). Despite its flaws, *Brittany Runs a Marathon* remains one of the best encapsulations I've seen of the things fat people—and fat women, in particular—settle for because we aren't taught to expect any better. It makes a sad kind of sense, really; how are we supposed to demand more from our friends, from our partners, from our bosses, from ourselves, when the world continually reminds us our bodies are obstacles, not vehicles?

I wish I'd known, back in the days when I feared fat more than anything, that the solution to this particular problem didn't lie in weight loss; after all, if I'd spent the past three-plus years of the COVID-19 pandemic recommitting myself to a strict diet and punitive exercise regimen instead of gaining weight and commencing the internal work necessary to start to be okay with it, I know with full certainty that I'd still be living in fear of gaining weight (or "the weight," as I so often called it, referring to the phantom accrual of pounds that had haunted me since middle school as if it were a real, tangible object living somewhere out there in the world, waiting for me). I'm glad I initiated the process of detaching exercise from size and, thus, my self-worth, but I wish I hadn't felt so alone as I was doing it; I wonder what my relationship with exercise could have looked like in my teens and early twenties if I'd seen more portrayals of active fat people in popular culture, presented without the underlying message that they were only as valuable as the weight they were able to lose.

As I adjusted to the significant weight gain that accompanied my last few years in Brooklyn, I started running less and less. In the past, my periods of falling out of the habit of physical activity had always coincided with my depressive, withdrawn, binge-heavy periods, but this time felt different. I wasn't quitting wholesale—I'd still go for at least one run per month, if only for the tiny pleasure of logging the excursion in my running app—but I slowly started to mix in other forms of exercise that were gentler on my knees, noting as I did so how judgmental I was of myself when it came to the process of moving my body. At first, the old maxim "If you don't sweat, it doesn't count" played on a loop in my head when I opted for a beginners' Yoga with Adriene class or headed out for a leisurely swim, but eventually, as I got more confident in the water and my bones got used to downward-dog pose, I started to notice that even exercise I hadn't chosen specifically for its calorie-burning potential had the capacity to strengthen my body and quiet my mind in a way I desperately needed.

By the time Natalie and I wedged our way into the over-stuffed, ten-year-old Honda Fit I'd bought from my cousin Tim and set out on the cross-country road trip that would deposit me in Austin in the summer of 2021, I weighed more than I ever had before. Yet—perhaps paradoxically to those who still insist obesity precludes the possibility of regular physical movement—I was more active than I'd been since the end of college, a time when I swam laps in the campus pool every few days and thought nothing of a five-mile round-trip bike ride through the woods to go pick up tampons and Pinnacle Whipped Cream Vodka from the Rite Aid in town. As Natalie and I made our way across the South in the scorching heat, driving for even longer stretches than we'd planned in order to avoid the effects of Hurricane Ida in New Orleans, I felt a strange buzzing in my limbs that I eventually identified as a bodily craving for movement. I'd yearned to run for miles back in LA when I was skinny and starving and always in search of a way to shed a few extra crucial pounds, but this felt like something else, a more primal urgency inside of me that I'd lost touch with somewhere around the time I first learned how to diet away my baby fat.

My notion of myself as inherently sedentary long preceded my fatness; in fact, it stretched all the way back to my babyhood, a time when—according to family lore—I learned to walk early but refused to actually do it for several years, instead waiting for someone to pick me up and ferry me to wherever it was I wanted to be. By the time I moved to Texas, though, leaving my treasured and hard-won Brooklyn social world behind to work remotely for *Vogue* from a one-bedroom apartment in Austin that I could actually afford to live in solo, I'd gotten used to getting exercise in some form at least three days a week, and even being cooped up in the car for seven days straight was enough to make my body demand its rightful share of movement. (What's "right" for me exercise-wise, it should be said, still varies greatly; there are weeks when I exercise five or six times and weeks when I manage to peel myself off the couch for only a single fifteen-minute walk to the coffee shop, but I finally trust myself and my body to find our way to some kind of equilibrium.)

I don't want to give the false impression that my current relationship with exercise is an uncomplicated one; I may not be running much anymore, but I can still find it within myself to dread swimming, yoga, hiking, kayaking, walking, and any other workout I do regularly until I'm actually in the process of doing it. There's a pleasant stillness, though, that reliably comes when I'm halfway through my set of laps at the YMCA or when I reach the point in my Yoga with Adriene video where my hips start to ache (despite Adriene's exhortation to "get in there, get a little juicy"). Ideas for stories that elude me during work hours often show up in my head in the middle of all this stillness, making me want to pause and grab a notebook, but I keep at it instead, gently pushing myself because I know that if I stop, it will be that much harder to start the next time—and I want to start the next time, to roll out my yoga mat or summit my favorite hiking trail or drive home from the pool with chlorine in my hair and the Chicks blasting on the radio. It took me so long to trust myself—to eat normally, to eat at all, to get outside when I'd rather stay in bed and binge—and now that I finally do, I want to honor the body I spent so long hating with the kind of movement that makes it feel good, whether it's a multiple-mile hike or a stoned, snail's-pace walk to pick up a latte.

In her 2021 book *Yoke: My Yoga of Self-Acceptance*, yoga practitioner, teacher, and writer Jessamyn Stanley talks about the freedom she felt when she first started doing yoga on her own at home, rather than in studio classes where she was often the only fat—let alone Black or queer—person present. "At home, everything was on the table," writes Stanley, adding: "I could wear my underwear, smoke weed, and share meditative breaths with my cat. It didn't matter that I only knew a few postures. Instead of going my usual route of obsessing over everything I *didn't* know, I focused all my energy on the eight to ten poses that I *did* know." When I'd occasionally gone to yoga classes back in LA, I'd panicked over whether I'd be able to hold myself up in crow pose and whether the instructor hated me for coming in three minutes late and—always, inevitably—how my body rated in comparison to the Lycra-clad ones stretching all around me, but when I started watching Stanley's YouTube tutorial videos at home in quarantine, I noticed how much of that anxiety and judgment was suddenly . . . gone.

My renewed interest in yoga over the past few years came partly from practicing alone (and, yes, often in my underwear with a joint in hand) in my bedroom, but I can recognize now that it also came from watching someone shaped like me move through the poses that had once seemed intimidating, presenting me with clear evidence that my body wasn't inherently incapable of performing these particular miracles. Nothing, though, has been more impactful in my exercise journey than working out with a fat trainer, as I started doing in the spring of 2022 when R.—the person I'd met on Twitter and started dating long-distance in the winter of my first year in Austin, with whom things unfolded in a way that felt more passionate yet infinitely more sane than any of my previous relationships—booked us a joint session with their friend Caroline, a comedy writer who'd gotten her personal-trainer certification during the pandemic.

Caroline was—and is—a brilliant trainer, bringing constant support and boundless creativity to every strength-training session (for that first one, she devised a whole workout plan themed around fictional journalists in rom-coms, because R. had told her what I did for a living), but the first thing I noticed about her was her body, somewhere close in size to mine and almighty-seeming as she led us through burpees and swung giant kettle-bells with ease in her pastel Girlfriend Collective athleisure. I'd barely ever seen other fat people in the exercise classes I'd taken up until then, let alone fat instructors, but I desperately wish that I had, because one workout with Caroline left me more simultaneously energized and at peace than I ever remembered feeling after exercise. We didn't talk about our bodies during the workout; instead, the three of us gossiped about TV and memes and LA queers we knew in common as we sweated and stretched on the studio mats—but it felt like something silent passed between us that day, a shared understanding of what it meant to move in a world that constantly told you exercise wasn't *for* people like you.

Jessie Diaz-Herrera, also known as @curveswithmoves on Instagram, knows plenty about helping people cultivate relationships with movement that aren't centered on weight loss. As a plus-size certified fitness instructor, she's used to working with clients who come in seeking to undo decades' worth of trauma around appearance, body size, and exercise, and she sees it as part of her mission to help them begin to untangle those complex associations. "It's so easy to go into a class as the only plus-size person there and immediately be like, *Oh God, am I going to enjoy myself? Are people going to be looking at me? Is this class going to be above my level?*" says Diaz-Herrera, adding: "There's definitely a sense of relief that I see when people come to a class with a plus-size instructor, but many of the people I train are coming from a place of having been burned before."

It's not hard for Diaz-Herrera to relate to her clients on issues of weight and self-worth, as she's dealt with them herself ever since she started dancing as a child. When she was only twelve, a ballet teacher instructed Diaz-Herrera to lose weight, leading her to cut out meals and eventually faint in dance class; she describes resenting her mother at the time for making her quit ballet after the fainting incident, but now, she says she's grateful to her for demonstrating clearly to her preteen daughter that it was not okay for her to be encouraged to harm or weaken herself. "That was definitely a really hard part of my life, and as a mom myself now, I'm learning that you have to ingrain those affirmations and let kids know they're amazing from the get-go, because building that self-confidence in them is so key," says Diaz-Herrera.

Diaz-Herrera began finding her way back to a joyful relationship with dance when she fell hard for hip-hop in college, telling me: "My body felt so good in dance, and then my body was deemed not good enough for dance, so it really took a lot for me to get myself back into dancing, even though I still held a lot of scrutiny around my body and dealt with dance costumes only coming in certain sizes, and stuff like that." It can be indescribably difficult to learn to place trust in exercise—as a habit, as a discipline, or even as a mental-health lifeline—when you still bear the emotional scars from a previously disordered relationship with dance or running or swimming or any other form of physical activity, but Diaz-Herrera's story is just one of the many that illustrate that it's possible—and infinitely worth the trouble—to begin the process of prying movement apart from self-image.

There are plenty of difficult things about exercising as a fat person—just ask anyone over a size 2XL or a D cup about their experience of trying to find workout clothes that fit properly, and you're sure to hear some war stories—but the thing that gets in my way most often as a fat runner, swimmer, hiker, and yoga practitioner isn't the world's judgment and size bias; it's the anxiety I place on *myself* about my own ability, sure every time I set out for a run or a trail hike that *this* will be the time I can't finish. I'm trying my best to recast this anxiety as a direct consequence of the fatphobia and ableism that growing up in aughts America inculcated in me, rather than any defect of mine. After all, my body still stores within it acute muscle memory of what it was like to propel myself through the Death Valley heat on an empty stomach in my days of caloric restriction, so I can't really blame it for not implicitly trusting me to give it what it needs. But it's a process, as they say, one that I really initiated in earnest only over the last two or three years of my life and don't anticipate myself being done with anytime soon.

As I write this, I can objectively recognize that I'm happier and more stable than I ever have been before in my life, but it's been difficult to make peace with the notion that even getting to the point where I am now—self-sufficient and employed full-time as a writer, with a wonderful partner who loves me and a wide group of family and friends I can always turn to for support—can't fix my lingering food and body issues for good. I'm loved and in love, writing things I care about for a living and building a life for my-self, and yet—*and yet*—I still binge sometimes, still spend money I don't have on massive orders of delivery food I don't really want and cancel plans the next morning when I wake up bleary-eyed and nauseous and unable to do more than lie prone on my sullied sheets, and regretting everything. The first time I exercise after a binge always feels miserable for the first few minutes, as though I'd undone all the good I'd done to and for my body merely by filling myself past the point of satiety yet again; I know intellectu-ally that that's not how it works, that I need and deserve to give myself credit for eventually changing the sheets and throwing out the binge-food remnants and getting out the door in my workout clothes and doing my best to right the ship, but knowing some-thing and feeling it are two different things.

I started keeping a binge log in January 2022 in the hazy, tear-ful aftermath of a particularly bad binge. I was in the process of putting together the proposal for the very book you're reading now, and although the prospect of writing openly about my experience with binge eating disorder should theoretically have been a liberating one, all it did was terrify me. I'd worked so hard for this opportunity, stringing together years' worth of "body beat" stories and researching disordered eating in my spare time (not, it should be said, the most upbeat of pursuits) and doing my best to write honestly—if only in my Notes app, for myself—about what it felt like to be a fat person trying to heal a fraught relationship with food, exercise, and body size, yet actually envisioning anyone reading a *memoir* about what I had to say on the topic filled me with the same fear I'd experienced when I'd been hired as an assistant on the Amazon show back in LA. I'd always expected that "getting my shit together," whatever that meant, would cure my bingeing, but the more I gained in life, the more I feared losing— and by then, the habit of using food to numb that fear was too deeply ingrained to fully excise.

My binge log is hard for me to look over, even with the benefit of a therapist and an ED-trained nutritionist now working in tandem to help me in my recovery from binge eating disorder. In the log, I note every single thing I eat during a binge, including any other factors that may have affected the experience—like being drunk or high—and my best shot at describing my mental state at the time (which, as I read over the document, often amounts to "anxious about X" or "depressed about X"; when it comes to mental illness, I'm nothing if not consistent). I'm proud of myself for recording my binges instead of letting them fade into the ether; I'm working so hard these days to extend myself grace and compassion for my binges, to forgive myself for yesterday even as I strive to do better today, and yet, when I total up how much time and money I've spent trying to push down my feelings with food, I can't help feeling bereft.

When I'm having a particularly hard time grappling with my recent history of binges, I try to remind myself to pull up the exercise log I started keeping on my Notes app in January 2021. I'd always liked the FitPoints aspect of Weight Watchers, in which you were given the option to trade exercise for extra calories, but I hated how tracking my exercise in the diet app seemed to rob it of what little intrinsic joy I took in it, so—copying something I'd seen a fat-positive fitness influencer do on Instagram—I created a system of recording and updating my physical activity that existed separately from my ongoing quest to lose weight. I wasn't ready to give up Weight Watchers or the diet-culture mentality behind it, but I knew by then that I simply felt better when I exercised, and I wanted to have a visual record of all my workouts so that when I inevitably hit a wall and felt incapable of getting back on the track or in the pool after a long period of sedentary bingeing, I'd have something concrete to show myself about just what my body had proved itself capable of.

I make a new exercise log every year, counting anything longer than a fifteen-minute walk toward my weekly total, and as I look back over all the exercise I've dutifully totaled over the past three years, I notice that there are only two or three weeks during all that time that don't contain at least one form of physical activity (and at least one of them came while I was recovering from COVID and discouraged from exercising). Running appears in my exercise log, as do yoga and swimming and the Zoom cardio class that Maya's sister Jackie taught us remotely for the first year of the pandemic, but plenty of entries simply read "17-minute walk home from bar" or "15-minute ocean swim" or "6-hour restaurant shift" (that last one cropping up frequently during the six months I spent hostessing at a French bistro on weekends during my first year in Austin). The still-disordered part of my brain might encourage me to count only intense, sweaty, "official" exercise toward my total, but I first initiated the log with the intention of noting *all* of the movement I engaged in from week to week, and all these years later, it still helps me to go back to the first item in my very first log—"24 min run around fort greene," logged on a random Wednesday—and think about all the adventures I've been strong enough to take my body on since then.

I don't expect my exercise regimen to "cancel out" my food issues anymore, but I'm also in no way done building a positive relationship with exercise; I'm proud of all the workouts I've logged over the past few years, but I still judge myself when a hike takes me twenty minutes longer than it did the previous week, or when I suddenly find myself exhausted halfway through a yoga video that usually leaves me feeling energized. These days, most of the work I do around movement and self-worth involves reminding myself that I don't have to make myself suffer—or, indeed, even engage in typical forms of exercise—in order to feel good in my body.

I do my best to devote most of my social-media usage to seeking out people who remind me of this truth, and one of my favorites is Fancy Feast, the Brooklyn-based burlesque performer and sex educator who boasts more than ten thousand followers on Instagram. That said, Fancy Feast is quick to note that her work doesn't revolve around internet validation: "I don't have social media outside of my burlesque persona, which makes decision-making a little easier in terms of not having to wonder, *Does this get presented or not? Is this going to be good for my brand or not?*" she says, adding: "My favorite thing about burlesque is that it is a continuation of the lives people live in their bodies; I love watching people tell stories with their bodies and find community around experiencing glamor and performing gender and addressing identity through performance in ways that are authored by the performers themselves."

Fancy Feast has spoken before—most notably in Leon Chase's 2017 documentary *Fancy Feast: The Fat Burlesque Dancer*—about the representational anxiety she occasionally feels as one of a mere handful of well-known fat performers in the burlesque space, telling Chase on camera: "I do feel the need to do well as a sort of ambassadorship on the behalf of fat girls everywhere. Which is a joy and a piece of shit burden." Ultimately, Fancy Feast is cognizant of what her act could mean to fat viewers who may never have watched someone who looked like them enact confidence and unabashed sexuality onstage before, telling me: "Burlesque was the first time I saw glamorous and exalted fat bodies out in the world. I had seen sexualized fat bodies in porn and stuff like that, but seeing those bodies being subjectified—rather than objectified—really feels quite revolutionary. I'm also interested in what exists for fat people beyond proving that they can be sexy. I try to think about: How else can I use the grammar of burlesque to challenge and start conversations?"

Burlesque performing isn't for everyone—neither are running or yoga or swimming or any other form of exercise, for that matter—but Fancy Feast hopes her relationship with bodily movement can inspire other fat people to claim the joy of physical activity for themselves: "In the times in my life where I've had a more difficult relationship with eating and movement," she says, "that negative self-talk can crowd out the ability to feel true pleasure and curiosity about art and my own life and the lives of others. My hope is that if people see me being loved and joyful and good at what I do, they can put down whatever pitchforks they're using to stab themselves down and just try to enjoy things and feel okay for at least a little bit of time."

As I write this, I am fatter than I've ever been, yet for one of the first times in my life, I'm also consistently exercising three to five times a week. What's more, I finally trust myself to keep working to create a relationship with movement that makes me feel mentally healthy and physically calm, regardless of the impact it has on the way I look—or doesn't. It took me a long time to feel the truth of what I'm about to say, but I'm saying it, because I wish I'd heard it and believed it earlier: there is nothing whatsoever about my fat body or yours that precludes the possibility of genuine joy brought about through whatever form of movement or interaction with the outside world you love most (which could be cardio or strength training or burlesque, yes, but could also be as simple as sitting outside on a blanket and letting the wind rustle through your hair). One day, I hope that should-be-basic statement will ring true to the many, many people who still desperately need to believe it.

Chapter 8

TASTE

Sometime in the quarantine-hazy days of April 2020, I lay sprawled across the guest bed at my dad's house and started making a Notes-app list of all the nonbinge-associated memories of eating that I could cling on to at that point in time. Frantically recorded and grammatically incorrect and increasingly random, the list ended up looking (in part) something like this:

hot dogs from rippers at rockaway

nora ephrons recipe for key lime pie

pear juice in rome, the kind from the carton

moms shepherds pie

the overly cinnamon y coffee eliza makes me in my big chipped white and gray mug tamar's panzanella

dad's broccoli a la emma

cadbury crunchie

tacos at mercado la paloma

blackberries i picked as a kid and melted w chocolate

The list went on for hundreds of entries after that, ultimately resembling nothing so much as the kind of lazily abstract poetry I had tried to pass off as my best work in any number of college creative-writing classes. (I'd tried my hand at fiction, hacking and clawing away at a set of linked stories for the better part of my junior year, but poetry always eluded me.) I'd gotten the idea to make the list from Alice, the first nutritionist I ever saw; we started meeting via Zoom about a month into quarantine, once I had well and truly got it through my head that I was alone with food for the foreseeable future, and although I desperately wanted to get better—to be the kind of person who could enjoy a good meal without pushing ever-forward to the place where it hurt—I resented the hell out of the person I'd found on ZocDoc to help me do just that.

Alice was a chirpy and reed-thin woman whose insistence on reexplaining portion sizes in all of our sessions made me feel (a) stupid and (b) insane, but I have to admit that the list she had recommended making was a good idea, even if I rarely looked at it. Alice wanted me to pull up the list on my phone whenever I felt out of control around food, but as time went on and pandemic restrictions abated and I recommended living a life out in the world again, I mostly forgot about it instead. I'd felt good about it while I'd written it, though; looking over at all the meals in my life I'd enjoyed enough to remember—from the In-N-Out fries dipped in a vanilla shake at Topanga State Beach to the condensed-milk-heavy iced coffee I'd downed in Hanoi that left me wired from sugar and caffeine to the chocolate mousse my parents had always let me order for dessert at the restaurant that had been our favorite when we'd lived in Rome—made me feel as though I had a relationship with food that existed beyond the binary confines of "eating too much" or "not eating enough."

I'm not sure when or how I (mostly) stopped being scared of food, but what I can say is that as of right now—August 19, 2023—I haven't dieted or consciously restricted my calories in over a year. I canceled my Weight Watchers subscription at least that long ago; my last binge was only last night, and I'm feeling as bruised and nauseous as I ever did in its aftermath, but intellectually, I know the two-month streak of abstinence that preceded it is still worth being proud of. My current nutritionist, Mia—the second one I ever saw, and the first one I learned enough from to make the astronomical out-of-pocket cost of the sessions feel worth it—reminded me of this in our last session, telling me for what must have been the dozenth time not to let any one slipup cancel out the strength and clarity it took to live so many days binge-free; after all, there were long stretches of my recent past when I could barely string a few days together without binge-ing, and if I don't acknowledge how hard I worked to overcome those times, I'm all the more at risk of repeating them.

If I'd been given that advice at another time in my life, or by someone other than Mia, I think I probably would have scoffed at it, unwilling as I was to display any of my probably obvious vulnerability around food. Throughout my early twenties, I read anything I could get my hands on about how other people ate, from Joan Didion's descriptions of protagonist Maria Wyeth's penchant for hard-boiled eggs in the 1970 novel *Play It as It Lays* to every single Grub Street Diet that *New York* magazine ever published; today, I still love descriptions of food in writing, but back then, I think I was just seeking a compass. I can see now that I gobbled up the details of other people's everyday food indulgences like the high-calorie baked goods and salty snacks I so rarely allowed myself outside of a binge context, desperately trying to understand how I should nourish myself when nobody was watching.

It's not that Mia's nutritional advice always works; she's not a magician, just the first actively fat-positive clinician I've ever encountered in my life (which, when you consider the institutionalized fatphobia that the medical profession is rife with, *can* feel a little bit like a magic trick). I trust Mia, but more important, I trust myself; I know I've fucked up with food before, but I also know that for each and every fuckup there's been a meal eaten with people I love, a recipe cooked to perfection, a post-binge morning when I got out of bed and washed my face and made coffee and recommitted to the ongoing project of living joyfully—or at least neutrally—in my body. (While the world might assume any number of things about my health from my current size, I know that my eating disorder thrived most during the time I spent enmeshed in the all-too-common diet-binge cycle, alternating binges with renewed commitment to Weight Watchers; I'm committed to not going back there, no matter how hard it is.) It still feels like I break that trust anew every time I stuff my body past its capacity, but I'm coming around to the idea that maybe the work I've done to try to heal my eating disorder isn't the kind of thing that can be undone; it's always there, in me, bobbing underwater like that old cliché about the ducks that appear placid on the surface while their webbed feet paddle away below to keep them afloat.

When I first read *Milk Fed*, Melissa Broder's 2021 novel about Rachel, a lapsed Jewish girl living in LA who worked on the fringes of Hollywood and tried to push down her emerging queerness with a laser-sharp focus on calorie restriction (um, hello), I couldn't shake the uncanniness of hearing someone else—even a fictional protagonist—describe the kind of mental arithmetic and constant self-monitoring that had defined my relationship with food for years. My heart soared when Rachel finally let herself eat to her heart's content at *shabbos* dinner with her secret girlfriend Miriam's family, exulting in Broder's description of the crispy, celery-stuffed roast chicken and the *tsimmes* and the challah—oh, the challah!—while simultaneously recalling the many Yom Kippur break-fasts I'd spent at my parents' friends' houses on one diet or other, studiously ignoring plates studded with H&H bagels, capers, tomato, and salty-fresh orange lox in favor of virtuously logging "2 pieces celery, half serving turkey meatloaf, ½ latke" into my Weight Watchers app. (Sidenote: Do you know how hard it is to eat *half* a latke?)

Ironically enough, it was during the High Holidays of 2021

that I found myself finishing *Milk Fed* for the first time, on a bench in Riverside Park with a cup of matzo ball soup from Zabar's in my hand. I'd made the trek to the Upper West Side with Maya and Kate so that Kate could take her yearly *You've Got Mail* homage photo at the Ninety-first Street Garden where Tom Hanks and Meg Ryan finally reunite (I wish I could tell my eighth-grade self that I would someday have friends who planned whole crosstown excursions around romantic comedies). Once the business of the day was completed, the girls set off to catch the train back to Brooklyn; I stuck around in the park, though, leafing through Broder's orange-bound book at hyper-speed as I tried to find out what happened to Rachel. Would she get better? Would she make a life with Miriam? Would food always be hard for her? It's not hard, now, to guess at the real motivation behind my rabid curiosity: Would food always be hard for *me*?

Once the sun began to set, I made my way back to Brooklyn, too, feeling the weight of the chocolate babka I'd picked up for my roommates through the thin fabric of my tote bag. When I got back to the apartment, though, nobody was home, which was rare in our chaotic but lively four-person setup. I felt depressed for a moment as I watched the light sink through the trees I could just barely glimpse out the window, but as I began pulling things out of my bag and putting them in their respective places—the leftover matzo ball soup in the fridge, the pierogi in the freezer, the blue-and-white-packaged babka in the bread box on the kitchen island—it dawned on me that I had the house to myself for one of the first times since I'd moved in three years prior. I doled out some soup and pierogi to myself, poured a glass of red wine, and sat on the couch eating and watching a rerun of *The Nanny*, exulting in my solitude instead of dreading it for once; I could put anything on the TV that I wanted, smoke weed in the living room, blast music or sit in silence, and still know people were eventually coming home to be with me, or at least with themselves in the same space as me.

The babka looming large over that night, thrumming with unrealized potential like Chekhov's proverbial gun; *Would I eat it? If so, how much? Would I finish it? Would anyone know? Where would I hide the packaging?* I remember cutting myself that first slice apprehensively, as though the loaf's binge potential could sneak up on me from behind; it had been a long time since I'd eaten dessert *stam*, "because because," rather than as part of a binge, and for once, the red wine and the bowl I'd smoked heightened my senses instead of dulling them. The thick ribbons of chocolate in the babka melted onto my tongue, followed by the soft caress of dough and the metallic-sharp flavor of the milk I chugged from one of my roommate Kristen's novelty mugs; the goodness hit me somewhere below my solar plexus but above my pelvis, traveling upward until I was almost lightheaded from how . . . well, *pure* the taste was. I'd spent so long harming myself with foods that looked and tasted just like this, but how could something so sweet—so alive—hurt me?

Of course, even in my sugar-and-carbs reverie, I knew that the babka on my plate certainly had the potential to hurt me, but I didn't let it—not that night, anyway. I ate one more slice and fell asleep easily, the way I almost never did at that point in my life, dreaming hazy dreams about Rachel and Miriam and Fran

Drescher and babka and pierogies and my own distant Jewish ancestors, none of whose first names I knew (although I did at least have a surname—Ratner—to use as a starting point if I ever wanted to learn more about the Russian Jews on my mom's side of the family, thanks to some Ancestry.com sleuthing my uncle had done a few years prior). I was the definition of a "cultural Jew," or so I told people—I'd been to temple only a few times, with family friends, and I'd spent those occasions counting the number of hats in the synagogue in a shameless imitation of Judy Blume's plucky tween protagonist in the 1970 novel *Are You There, God? It's Me, Margaret*—but Jewish food, and all that I associated with it, felt like the definition of what my body craved and my mind feared. I wanted it, and I wanted to let myself want it; food was one way my people had cared for one another throughout time and tragedy, and the prospect of continuing to deny myself forever was starting to feel almost worse than the denial itself.

Self-denial isn't something I'm particularly interested in organizing my life around anymore, yet as I write this, I'm cognizant of the fact that I'm out of step with the times, as we're living through yet another "thin-is-in" cultural moment heralded by the mass-market availability of weight-loss drugs like Ozempic, Wegovy, and Mounjaro. These brand-name versions of the anti-diabetic medication semaglutide were developed in 2012, but in 2021, the FDA approved them for weight management in adults with obesity who had at least one comorbidity; the "Ozempic craze" that soon followed in Hollywood, though, was mostly spurred by people who did not have obesity looking to arm themselves with a secret weapon against the perennial problem of hunger. Elon Musk was an early adopter of the now-prevalent trend of using Ozempic for weight loss, posting to Twitter about his fondness for the drug in October 2022, but Ozempic's mainstream popularity can largely be attributed to TikTok, where the #Ozempic hashtag has now accrued over a billion views.

The February 27, 2023, issue of *New York* magazine is one whose cover I can still vividly recall; "Bon Appétit," read a bold-typed white caption superimposed over an image of a fork stabbing the hollow plastic part of a syringe. Inside the issue was features writer Matthew Schneier's cover story on Ozempic, which featured a range of Ozempic users' least politically correct admissions about the various motives behind their use of a costly and side-effect-heavy drug that, as Schneier wrote, provided an "effortless, near-instant fix." In Schneier's story, an actress on Ozempic testifies to surviving on "one and a half meals a day," while another woman confesses she'd maybe rather risk thyroid cancer than give up the injectable she now relies on to lose weight; if you live with an eating disorder, or maybe even if you don't, it's hard not to get triggered reading these pseudonymous interviewee's casual admittances of everything they're willing to give up in pursuit of thinness.

Here's what really bothers me about the weight-loss-drug craze: if Ozempic had been approved by the FDA for bariatric use at any point in my teens or early twenties, I'm confident that I would at least have tried to get my hands on it, and—given the freedom with which the ZocDoc-sourced, mildly shady doctor I saw back then prescribed me Adderall I didn't really need—I probably would have succeeded, even during the periods when I weighed the least. Back then, I saw fat as the enemy, the villain waiting in the wings to condemn me to a life of insecurity and loneliness; if you'd told me that there was a medication on the market that would simply zap my stubborn, persistent hunger, my oh-so-unsightly longing for food, I would have regarded it as a miracle cure for everything I perceived to be so very wrong with me, and I probably wouldn't have stopped until I found someone to provide me with it.

The idea of trading everything I've accumulated over the past few years—my fatness, yes, but also my taste for food, my interest in cooking, my ability to relish a good meal at least some of the time—for thinness now feels like the ultimate Faustian bargain, but I know that the "Ozempic craze" might have sucked me up into its wake if it had taken root even just a few years earlier, before I'd had the benefit of enough time and regular therapy to begin to deprioritize weight loss. I also know there are people for whom weight-loss medications like Ozempic and Wegovy provide a huge benefit, and I don't want to pass judgment on anyone's health regimen or individual relationship with food, but I worry that drugs like these provide a quick fix to the messy and often lifelong problem of learning to live in a changeable and desirous human body. Where would I be now if I'd gotten accustomed to spending $900 a month—essentially a second rent—on weight-loss drugs in 2017, instead of finding my way to a twelve-step food group and starting Abilify and moving to New York and reading Roxane Gay and initiating the process of learning to occupy space in my own body?

It's taken me years to be able to say this, but as I sound it out in my head, it feels true; I mostly like my hunger. I've grown accustomed to it, and I learn its contours every day when I wake up and try to figure out whether cereal or a big, greasy breakfast burrito or a green juice or just coffee would feel best in my stomach. I try to take the advice I once got from writer and curve model Kendra Austin, who has written extensively about her own experiences living with disordered eating, to "eat dessert every day"; or, at least, to eat dessert whenever I want it, especially when I'm feeling bad about the wanting itself. (When the old mental reflex to "just stick some grapes in the freezer!" or "just pick up some Halo Top!" goes off in my head, that's when I know I *really* need dessert—as in, actual dessert, not diet ice cream that tastes like Splenda-sweetened snow.) I used to think of my hunger as something feral, out of control—an untamed animal who needed to be sedated as much as possible, lest it rise up and maul me—but now, I'm trying to see it as more of a kindly invited guest, someone whose preferences and tastes I let guide me without overwhelming me entirely.

The idea of becoming constitutionally uninterested in food no longer holds the kind of power that it once did; I still hate myself in the aftermath of my binges, but I can recognize that they're much less frequent than they used to be, and more to the point, I know they don't represent the sum total of my relationship with food. I'm not willing to give up the oceanic chill of the oysters R. and I sucked down on our first date with our feet *almost* touching under the table, or the comfort of a steaming bowl of pho eaten alone with a good book at my favorite Vietnamese lunch spot in Austin, or the warmth of the loaf of challah just out of the oven that I spent hours braiding into a six-strand twist last Rosh Hashanah. I want to learn to live in harmony with my appetite, not ditch my doctor (who, the last time I saw her, officially confirmed for me that weight-loss drugs weren't an ideal choice for someone with my ED history) and find one willing to help me chemically overwhelm it entirely.

I wish I could say I felt this way—confident in my size, skeptical of diet culture, unwilling to prolong my near-lifelong obsession with achieving maximum thinness—100 percent of the time, but unfortunately, that's not true. When I hear stories about dramatic celebrity slim downs or watch friends be praised by people I don't like for looking "so good!" after a bout of stomach flu, I'm still not immune from wondering if I should be focusing the majority of my energy on losing weight, too (no matter how deeply I'm starting to understand that weight loss isn't the problem for me; it's a distraction from the problem, a means of controlling my outside appearance so I don't have to focus on what's going on inside me). When those worries crop up, I do my best to feed myself compassionately, with good, nourishing food that I actively enjoy, of course, but also with renewed attention to the work of people who remind me how many different ways there are to be alive and eating—joyfully, voraciously, and curiously—in the world today.

One of those people is Bettina Makalintal, now a senior reporter for *Eater* who has previously written for *Bon Appetit* and *Vice*. Makalintal's food writing is both sanguine and genuinely challenging in its examination of the food world, but it's her cooking-archive Instagram account @crispyegg420 ("no recipe just vibes," as she describes it) that I turn to most often when I need a reminder of how far I've come from the LA days when I lived primarily on binge food, RXBARs, and stomach-roiling waves of unmedicated anxiety; still, even someone as intimately involved with food on a personal and professional level as Makalintal isn't necessarily immune from the pressures imposed by diet culture. "I sometimes wonder if I like cooking because I like food, or because it feels like an acceptable way to have a relationship with food and also have the body that I have," Makalintal tells me, adding: "I wonder if I fell into [food] as an interest because it seemed like a way to have power over this thing that I felt I had a bad relationship with."

Makalintal is just one of the many food professionals I've spoken to in the course of my career who struggle with some aspect of disordered eating and/or body dysmorphia, another of whom is Shaina Loew-Banayan, chef and owner of the James Beard Award–winning Cafe Mutton in upstate New York. The food that Loew-Banayan and their wife, also named Bettina, serve out of their small, wood-paneled restaurant on Columbia Street in Hudson is equally nourishing and creative, and the same might be said of their writing style, which they displayed in their 2022 memoir *Elegy for an Appetite*. As I read the book, I was struck by the way Loew-Banayan characterized their choice to pursue work in restaurant kitchens as a means of distraction from the gnawing, ever-present hunger that their eating disorder had instilled in them early on in their life. Loew-Banayan allows their delight in food to coexist (if somewhat uneasily) alongside their fear of it, capturing the two opposing approaches in poetic run-on sentences like: "We ate bone marrow with challah and matzoh ball soup at two in the morning. The following day, back on my hunger."

I, too, know intimately what it feels like to chase positive food experiences with negative ones. I've gone from relishing a good meal to overstuffing my body with its fridge-chilled leftovers more times than I can count, and the juxtaposition always feels extra-painful, a scarlet F scrawled on a report card that seems to cancel out the A you'd earned the day before. I do, however, think that food can offer a kind of antidote to the pain that bingeing can unleash on my body (a pain that's grown steadily worse as I've gotten older; back in my late teens and early twenties, I could and did binge for days on end without too much physical distress, but now that I've passed the age-thirty mark and my binges have gotten more infrequent, a single one is capable of sidelining me for the better part of a week as I struggle to calm my aching stomach).

These days, I'm doing my best to, in Loew-Banayan's memorable words, not get "back on my hunger"—or, in other words, starve—after a binge. I buy frozen pork-and-ginger soup dumplings by the boxful when I go to Trader Joe's, knowing through experience that their comforting mix of protein and broth will be the only thing I'll be remotely in the mood to eat when I wake up nauseous in sheets stained with food crumbs and my own sweat. This is what "self-care" means to me these days; not sheet masks and bubble baths, but stocking my freezer with food

I can have ready in five minutes while I'm desperately trying to regain my equilibrium the day after a late night of cramming Papa John's pizza or grocery-store ice cream into my mouth. In LA, I stock up on frozen kimchi buns at the Korean grocery store a few miles from R.'s house, hoping the starch and brine will help speed my recovery, and when I'm feeling *truly* incapable of eating after a binge, I fix myself tea with lemon and as much honey as I want, which hasn't yet gotten old to me, used as my brain still is to measuring out high-calorie sweets in painstaking teaspoonfuls. In these small ways, I do my best to be a friend to myself, not an enemy; I want to meet myself with generosity in the aftermath of pain, not compound it by refusing to give my body the rest and fuel it's begging me for.

When I started cooking real meals for myself sometime in the middle of my three-year stretch of time in LA, I was hesitant and skittish in the kitchen, even with a bounty of *Bon Appétit* and *New York Times* Cooking recipes to guide me. Recipes were the only way I trusted myself to actually execute a full, photo-worthy meal without bingeing on its component parts, but even when I did everything completely by the book, things didn't usually turn out great; I can recall the strangely lumpy sweet-potato stew and execrable attempt at *bánh xèo* (the shrimp crepes I'd soothed myself with as I rapid-cycled between mania and misery on a 2017 trip to Vietnam, shortly before I received my bipolar diagnosis) with some degree of affection now, but when I sweated over the stove all night in the tiny kitchen of the squat, stucco-walled Virgil Village apartment I briefly shared with Eliza—only to have my great attempt at meal-prepping for the week come out lousy—I would boil over with shame, sure that my failure reflected a larger inability to wrangle food onto my side.

I felt so deeply judged by people's perfect desk-lunch and dinner-out Instagrams in the years when my eating disorder was at its peak, and even now that I'm healthier and happier in every conceivable way, the same insecurities still crop up at times (most often when I've skipped one too many therapy sessions or haven't made the time to exercise or cook for myself in a while). Even someone as online-food-savvy as Makalintal understands this feeling, telling me: "Sometimes I don't cook and I'll just eat a bunch of vegetarian chicken nuggets, but I know the desire to cook is always going to come back to me. I try not to force it, and just accept that sometimes my food isn't going to be creative, or it's going to be ugly, or whatever. That's just part of the process, and I know that it's always going to be balanced out with another period of feeling like, 'Oh man, I just left the farmers market and I can't wait to cook with these beans or this eggplant.'"

There are plenty of weeks when I, too, show up at the farmers market with my baseball cap on and my tote bag tucked under my arm, ready to chat up vendors, sample toothpick-stabbed bites of produce, and find a use for the beets or kale or tomatoes I buy that night in the kitchen, with a candle lit and the Os Mutantes album *Tecnicolor* (my go-to cooking music) blaring in the background, using knowledge accrued from years' worth of strictly following recipes in order to freestyle a little with my miso or balsamic vinaigrette or fish sauce.

Conversely, there are probably just as many weeks when I exist on a loose patchwork of takeout, frozen Trader Joe's fare, and meals out at restaurants. Feeding myself on the fly like this definitely makes me more susceptible to bingeing, but the frustration of my eating disorder lies at least partially in the fact that there have been too many farmers market–going, meal-cooking weeks to count where I've *still* binged, even after nourishing myself healthfully and deliciously with a reasonable serving of whatever food I'd been craving. (Recovery isn't an exact science, something I should know by now but have to remind myself of anew each time I reset the clock after a long stretch of promising abstinence.)

To be a thin person perennially engaged in the Sisyphean task of avoiding food is more or less unremarkable in our society; when I stream old episodes of the aughts comedies I grew up watching, I'm grimly aware of how many jokes center on ultra-slender female characters' bizarre relationships with food, perhaps best encapsulated by Courteney Cox's character on *Cougar Town* habitually sucking on chocolates for a mere three seconds before spitting them out. What really seems to freak people out, though, is being confronted with the living fact of a fat person who *doesn't* fear food, or who at least doesn't constantly make a show out of fearing it. There was infinitely more cultural space for me to hate myself out loud when I was thin than there is, even now, for me to appreciate my appetite and my body as a fat woman, but the flip side is, I'm less worried about taking up space (physically, professionally, interpersonally, and otherwise) than I ever was when my main concern in life was being able to fasten a pair of size twenty-five jeans over my hips in the Cross-roads dressing room.

I still read Grub Street Diets hungrily now that I've learned how to food shop, cook, and eat in a way that mostly makes me feel good, but it's out of genuine interest, not despera-tion; I love knowing how other people feed themselves, what kind of desk lunches and leftover dinners they put together just for themselves. Possibly my favorite piece of food writing ever published, though, is a *Guernica* essay written by the au-thor Carmen Maria Machado in 2019 and titled "The Trash Heap Has Spoken," in which she gives a characteristically el-oquent voice to the subversive glee of being fat and relishing food: "I take second helpings, thirds. I order appetizers and des-serts. I get excited about homemade pasta and pork belly and chocolate cake and dirty martinis and bowls of pickled things. Sometimes when I talk about food, people around me laugh with surprise. Subconsciously, I think, they're not expecting it; they're expecting restraint, apology. I refuse to give it to them."

Sometimes it feels like I expend most of my energy trying to feed myself with this degree of jubilance—not, of course, that Machado's or anyone else's relationship with food is easy 100 per-cent of the time, but I desperately want to model for other people that it's possible to be as big as I am at my current weight (or far bigger) and still nurture a connection with and passion for food. Every time I get the buttery croissant and latte I really want at the coffee shop instead of grimly ordering a banana and a cup to go with skim milk, or refill my plate at Thanksgiving in blithe defiance of the disapproving eyes trained on me, I can feel the cumulative pain of all the years I spent wishing desperately to shrink myself; I honor that smaller, scared, sad version of me with each bite. *Just because we're fat,* I imagine myself self-righteously lecturing a horde of my fellow over-size-eighteen beauties in some conference room somewhere, *does not mean we owe the thin people in our lives dry salads and performative self-hatred and "No thanks, I'm on another diet" demurrals. We do not have to eat—or not eat—in the way they expect us to. We don't have to be afraid just because they are.*

I know, though, that yelling at people to accept themselves from behind a lectern or in an Instagram story or a TikTok doesn't generally tend to help them do it, so I try to content myself with eating exactly when and what I want in public as often as I can, hoping that my friends or colleagues or younger cousins who might not even know how desperately they need to see examples of happy, fat people out in the world will witness firsthand that there's nothing to be feared from following your hunger (even if it means gaining weight). I feel infinitely more awake and present in my life now than I ever did when I was thin, but for some reason, it's not enough for me just to sit with that truth; I'm still angry for all the years I felt otherwise, and some part of me wants to shout it from the rooftops or go door-to-door proselytizing so the disordered eaters who "still suffer"—as we used to put it in my twelve-step food group—will see it's possible.

Luckily, I'm far from alone in the ongoing project of attempting to nurture and display a positive relationship with food as a fat person. Makalintal, too, refuses to cede to the societal pressure to exist on low-calorie scraps for the sake of appearances, telling me: "I am an inherently stubborn person, and I think food is one of those areas where I just don't want to make concessions with my joy. It's one of those things that is so reliable to me for enjoyment, both in eating but also in the planning and the process of cooking; it's a space where I'm glad I get to exert my stubbornness. I don't want to cave in to all these things I hear other people say; yes, I feel body anxiety and I feel those pressures about what I should look like, but at the end of the day, I know what makes me happy and it's going to the grocery store and buying this thing or that thing and being really excited about it. I wouldn't trade any of that for the hypothetical pleasure that I might get out of enjoying food less."

I never expected to find myself saying this, but as I write this, I'm a Los Angeles resident once again; I repacked my trusty Honda Fit and made the move back to California in June 2023, after a year of dating R. long-distance. The possibility of R. and me living near each other in a city brimming with queer and trans communities and constantly illuminated by sunshine had thrilled me ever since we'd begun to talk about it a few months into our relationship (insert U-Haul joke here), but I needed a while to mull over the move before eventually deciding that I was ready to return to the place where some of my lowest lows had taken place. I've been here for just over three months now, and it's not perfect, nor am I perfect in it—I still binge sometimes, still lie, still hide and evade and obscure the truth of my suffering—but I'm learning to do all of that less as I adjust to a life lived within the immediate orbit of my first-ever serious partner, who just so happens to be a food writer—and who has taught me more than I could ever have imagined about what it means to have a truly generative connection to—and relationship with—food.

When I first met R. in the winter of 2021, they were working on a piece for the *Los Angeles Times* about the Mandarin Man, a Chinese immigrant who'd fled his home during the Cultural Revolution and now owned a family-run orchard in Chino Hills that grew tiny, impossibly sweet Kishu mandarin oranges; when I drove out to LA for a visit in November 2022, they sent me off at the month's end with a kiss and a Ralph's grocery bag packed to the brim with Kishus. I feasted on my bright orange bounty for the entirety of my road trip back to Austin, finding stray dark-green leaves from the Kishus' stems scattered on the floor and seats of my car for months afterward (and catching myself smiling in the rearview mirror every time I unearthed another one). I don't tell R. everything about my eating disorder as it exists today, but I tell them a lot—more than I've ever told anyone else—and there's a humiliating kind of freedom in talking to someone about it, in not being alone with my shame.

I can see now that the fear I felt throughout quarantine about going out into the world and attempting to date at my new size was my brain's sad attempt to protect me from rejection, because for years—even when I was thin—rejection and avoidance were the main themes of my romantic encounters. I refused to date when I was closeted and pursued too hard once I came out, chasing people who obviously didn't have the emotional bandwidth to give me what I needed, and then blamed my body when things didn't work out instead of acknowledging that I had some serious work to do in the emotional-growth department. In R., for the first time, I found a partner who made me feel secure instead of anxious in my attachment (or, at least, these were the words that the dog-eared copy of *Attached* I'd found on the street in Brooklyn encouraged me to apply to my relationship); from the beginning, they celebrated my fat body so enthusiastically and naturally that it was a little infectious, allowing me to see myself the way they saw me.

The first gift R. ever sent me, back when we were still new and giddily figuring out the contours of a long-distance relationship that stretched from Austin to Los Angeles, was a crop top so tiny that when I first unwrapped it, I thought it was a scarf. *That won't fit*, the old familiar demon voice in my brain cautioned once I figured out that it was a shirt, but it did: it was a deceptively stretchy size 2XL, painted in a patchwork of my favorite colors by a friend of R.'s who crafted gorgeous handmade clothes in a wide variety of sizes out of her studio in LA. The stretch marks on my waist and hips were on full display when I wore the shirt, a mass of purple, pink, and red claiming vibrant space against my pale skin, but I tried not to care—and even found myself (mostly) succeeding. I put the shirt on with my best white mom jeans, my pink sunglasses, and a pair of Crocs and studied myself in the filthy mirror in the bedroom of my apartment in Austin, trying my best to hear R.'s voice in my head before I even sent them a selfie: *You look hot.*

It's so tempting to me to leave my story there, on a high note of love and sex appeal and self-compassion learned via osmosis from a partner who truly cares for me, but to do so would be to give my life the glossy sheen of a rom-com edit instead of acknowledging the harsh truth that the ongoing work of recovering from my eating disorder has been long, arduous, and often lonely. I didn't magically stop harming myself with food once I fell in love, and even now—immersed as I am in the joy of building a life in LA with R.—I'm aware that I alone have to keep "doing the work," as much as I hate that euphemism, in order to achieve my goal of reducing my binges and stringing together ever-longer stretches of abstinence. (I no longer hold myself to the promise that I'll quit forever someday, knowing through experience that the idea of never bingeing again immediately makes the scarcity-attuned part of my brain panic; instead, my treatment plan for the last few years has centered on harm reduction, i.e., fewer and less-intense binges.)

Today, I sometimes look at my friends and colleagues in their early twenties—some struggling with the same food-sex-and-love-shaped burdens I did, some with radically different ones—and think: *I'll never say this out loud to you, because it's condescending, but time will pass and the pain will lessen and you will start to like yourself, at least a little bit.* My lows still feel pretty damn low sometimes—I'm trying with every bite to redefine my relationship with food into an overall-positive one, and the frustration of that struggle is ongoing—but I live a full life inside of, in spite of, or, fuck it, maybe even *because* of my "full-figured" (or, as I'm learning to be comfortable saying without apology, "fat") body. I'm trying my best, and now—as in, *right now*, as I sit here writing this on a hot September day in LA in an all-day lesbian bar that didn't exist the last time I lived here, pickled remnants of a chicken sandwich beside me and a milky cold brew in hand—I'm trying to let the trying be enough.

I didn't come up with the idea for this hybrid memoir-in-interviews solely in an attempt to heal my food wounds (although

I would probably have been willing to try it if I'd thought it would have worked, desperate as I was in 2021 to find any kind of escape hatch out of my binge eating and the chaos it seemed to unleash on my life), but I don't think there's a version of this book that exists without me first finding my way to some kind of fragile peace around my own body size and hunger. I wish desperately that I could tell every compulsive eater out there exactly how I did this—I used to rail against eating-disorder narratives in which getting better just "happened," as though it weren't sometimes a minute-by-minute, knockdown, drag-out fight for me just to get through the day without bingeing. But then I remember: I don't entirely know the how, myself. Or maybe that's not quite right; maybe the answer is that there's not just one answer, as annoyingly mystical as that sentence may sound.

I know that starting to do steady work in a field I cared about helped, as did a proper mental-health diagnosis and medication, as did surrounding myself with friends in New York, as did coming out and falling in real, reciprocated love and finding movement that satisfied me and taking true pleasure in food after a lifetime of denial. I'm fat now, there's that; I wasn't, five years ago. I'm also content with my life and my choices and the way I move through the world in a way I've never been. Is it because I'm fat? That doesn't quite feel right, although it's not *not* related to gaining weight and learning to live with it, in it, instead of in its shadow. Maybe gaining weight helped, but with the benefit of hindsight, I can see the obvious truth that I would have ridiculed five years ago: so did growing up. What a lucky thing to get to do.

ACKNOWLEDGMENTS

Thank you—first and foremost—to every member of the extended Specter/Stanley/Linfield clan. Nobody wants a memoirist in the family, and you've all dealt with it with generosity, humor, and grace. I love you all endlessly.

I owe more than I could ever express to my editor, Rachel Kambury, whose wisdom and empathy are matched only by her commitment to justice in all its forms. A good chunk of the writing of this book took place during the 2022–2023 Harper-Collins Union strike that Rachel helped lead, and I'll never forget watching her and her colleagues walk the picket line in the cold and rain for months to fight for a more inclusive and equitable vision of their industry. This book, and publishing as a whole, are infinitely better off because of Rachel.

My agents, Natalie Edwards and Allison Hunter of Trellis Literary, are two of the most thoughtful, creative, and relentlessly encouraging people I've ever worked with. (Special shoutout to the newly arrived Caroline Joan Hunter; baby's first acknowledgments mention?) Thank you to everyone at Trellis and HarperCollins for the labor and care you put into this project.

This book wouldn't exist without the generosity and openness of the people who consented to share their experiences with food, fatness, disordered eating, and healing in its chapters; thank you to Kendra Austin, Stephanie Covington Armstrong, Jessie Diaz-Herrera, Fancy Feast, Sabrina Imbler, Aiyana Ishmael, Leslie Jamison, Dani Janae, Isle McElroy, Marisa Meltzer, Virginia Sole-Smith, and Virgie Tovar for your invaluable input.

Thank you to everyone at *Vogue*—especially my past and present editors Jessie Heyman, Marley Marius, Chioma Nnadi, Chloe Schama, and Estelle Tang—for their constant support of my work, and thank you to all my Condé United union colleagues for showing up every day to make our workplace better.

I have the greatest friends in the world, and I wouldn't have been able to take on the project of excavating my often-painful history with food and weight over these past few years without their encouragement. Daniella Acker, Eliza Blum, Gavin Mead, Brett Miller, Natalie Reneau, and Rebecca Saltzman have steadily loved me, counseled me, and roasted me since we were eighteen-year-old idiots smoking weed in Ohio cornfields. Maya Kosoff and Kate Lindsay helped me find a version of New York that fit me (and made me laugh constantly via group text along the way). Beth Garrabrant, Amalie MacGowan, Gus Stanley, and Mickey Stanley made Austin feel like home. Jett Allen, Caroline Anderson, Dana Calvo, Nor Chang, Mads Gobbo, Lynn Hong, Jazmine and Gabe Kanengiser, Miles Klee, Lauren Kop, AC

Acknowledgments

Lamberty, Brent Lawson, Alana Levinson, Ruth Madievsky, Julie Mandel-Folly, Hannah Murphy, Teddy Pozo, Li Sanchez, Daniel Spielberger, and Julia Wick are my LA family, and I couldn't ask for a better one. Tamar Adler provided a crucial early read of this book, and I'm nearly as grateful for that as I am for her loyal friendship (not to mention her stellar recipe for carrot-top pesto).

R.: You are the sweetest gift I have ever received. Thank you for sharing your life (and your laptop charger) with me. I love you.

SUGGESTED FURTHER READING

Landwhale by Jes Baker

Milk Fed by Melissa Broder

Pleasure Activism: The Politics of Feeling Good by adrienne maree brown

Empty: A Memoir by Susan Burton

Dead Weight: Essays on Hunger and Harm by Emmeline Clein

Not All Black Girls Know How to Eat: A Story of Bulimia by Stephanie Covington Armstrong

Hunger: A Memoir of (My) Body by Roxane Gay

What We Don't Talk About When We Talk About Fat by Aubrey Gordon

Lessons from the Fat-O-Sphere: Quit Dieting and Declare a Truce with Your Body by Kate Harding and Marianne Kirby

Belly of the Beast: The Politics of Anti-Fatness as Anti-Blackness by Da'Shaun L. Harrison

The Recovering: Intoxication and Its Aftermath by Leslie Jamison

Heavy: An American Memoir by Kiese Laymon

This Is Big: How the Founder of Weight Watchers Changed the World (and Me) by Marisa Meltzer

Fat and Queer: An Anthology of Queer and Trans Bodies and Lives, ed. Miguel M. Morales, Bruce Owens Grimm, and Tiff Joshua TJ Ferentini

Fat Talk: Parenting in the Age of Diet Culture by Virginia Sole-Smith

Yoke: My Yoga of Self-Acceptance by Jessamyn Stanley

Fearing the Black Body: The Racial Origins of Fat Phobia by Sabrina Strings

The Body Is Not an Apology: The Power of Radical Self-Love by Sonya Renee Taylor

You Have the Right to Remain Fat by Virgie Tovar